Dr. Malhot

Step by

Anaesthesia in Obstetrics and Gynaecology

To
The patients who have taught us how to best care
for them, with the hope that we will remember the
lessons of the past and recognise the
lessons of the future

The pregnant patient presents a unique "two- in-one" situation for the anaesthesiologist; what happens to the mother has a bearing on her unborn child; also the foetus produces a whole gamut of physiological changes in the mother, which have important anaesthetic implications. Anaesthetic drugs and techniques affect both the uterus and the placenta—the link between the mother and the unborn child; the resultant changes can retard placental exchange of essential nutrients. These and other considerations unique to the pregnant state have been very well elucidated in this hand-book. The editors deserve a pat on the back for presenting an absorbing overview of the problems faced on the obstetric floor and their solutions.

RM Malhotra MBBS FICS
Prabha Malhotra MBBS DGO
Consultant Obstetricians
and Gynaecologists
Agra

Preface

The role of the anaesthesiologists in obstetric practice
has been redefined as advances in reproductive
medicine have improved obstetric outcome in women
despite significant systemic diseases and advancing
age. Today anaesthesiologists play an active and
important role in labour and delivery suites. Not only
they provide anaesthesia and analgesia but they are an
integeral part of the team of physicians who care for
the high risk pregnant patient. Keeping this in mind,
emphasis has been placed on management of high risk
parturient.

Previously "labour pain" was an accepted fact, but
in today's informed world, it is common knowledge
that safe and effective means are now available to
reduce labour discomfort. The obstetrician and patients
today, do not seek "anaesthesia" but demand only
"analgesia", be able to ambulate and also actively
participate in the birthing experience. The use of
neuraxial techniques and drugs described in the text,
address this new demand.

The information provided in chapters on HIV
positive parturient, medicolegal issues and practice
guidelines of obstetric anaesthesia, is likely to come
handy to the anaesthesiologists and obstetricians.

This hand book is designed to be a readily accessible
and accurate source of information on obstetric

anaesthesia for practicing anaesthesiologists, anaesthesia residents and "interested" obstetricians. We hope it will serve its purpose well.

Narendra Malhotra
Jaideep Malhotra

Acknowledgements

I am thankful to Prof. BL Gupta, Ex-Professor and Head, Department of Anaesthesiology, SN Medical College and Hospital, Agra who besides being my teacher has been my "guardian angel". His wisdom, guidance and love inspired me and helped to shape me into the person I am today.

To my parents, from whom I imbibed the virtues of honest, hard work and who taught me to love to learn, I am grateful.

I am thankful to Dr. Narendra Malhotra and Jaideep Malhotra for their constant encouragement which made it possible to write this piece of text.

I am extremely grateful to my wife Ranju and sons Rahul and Rajat whose constant support I rely on and count on so heavily.

Vinay Tewari

Acknowledgements

I am thankful to my mentor Dr Baljit Singh, Ex-Professor and Head, Department of Anaesthesia, Govt. Medical College, Patiala and Rtd DRME, Punjab, who taught me insight of anaesthesiology, think rationally, decision making, anticipate problems and plan in difficult situations.

I am also thankful to Dr Narendra Malhotra and Dr. Jaideep Malhotra for inspiring and constantly guiding me to write this book.

I am thankful to my mother and my son Nikhil who have supported and spared their time to complete this book.

Last but not the least I owe special thanks to my better half Dr Suman who always stood with me in all my endeavours.

PL Gautam

Contents

Section 5: Critical Care in Obstetrics

Section 6: Miscellaneous

SECTION 1

INTRODUCTION

Chapter 1

Anaesthesia Work Station Check Up

Anaesthesia equipment is used to deliver oxygen, nitrous oxide and inhalation anaesthetics and to control ventilation. Several monitors are used to observe the function of the system, to detect equipment failures and to provide information about the patient. Before using the equipment, it should be checked to rule out any malfunction and to ensure adequate back up measures are available, if needed.

For the First Case of the Operation List

1. Check that the anaesthetic machine is connected to the power supply (if necessary) and switched on. Pay attention to any information on the machine, particularly servicing details.
2. Check oxygen analyser is present, turned on, checked and calibrated.
3. Check gas supply connections.
   - Identify the gases being supplied by pipeline; confirm by a 'tug test' that the gas supply terminal is connected to the appropriate pipeline.
   - Check that the anaesthetic machine is connected to a supply of oxygen and that an adequate supply of oxygen is available from a reserve oxygen cylinder.
   - Check that adequate supplies of other gases (such as nitrous oxide and air) are available and connected.
   - Check that all pipeline pressure gauges in use indicate 400 kPa.

4. Check the operation of flow meters.
   - Ensure smooth operation of the flow control valve and check that the bobbin moves freely throughout its range.
   - Check oxygen failure device.
   - Check the operation of the emergency oxygen bypass control.
5. Check the vapouriser(s).
   - Ensure that each vapouriser is adequately filled but not over-filled.
   - Ensure that each vapouriser is correctly seated on the back bar.
   - Check the vapouriser for leaks, both in "on" and "off" positions. Turn the vapouriser off.
   - A leak test should be performed immediately after changing any vapouriser.
6. Check the breathing system.
   - The system should be visually inspected for correct configuration.
   - A pressure leak test should be performed on the breathing system by occluding the patient port and compressing the reservoir bag.
   - Bain's circuit should be checked for integrity of inner tube using Venturi's principle. Press oxygen flush; with this the reservoir bag should collapse indicating generation of negative pressure.
   - The correct operation of unidirectional valves should be checked if closed circuit or circle absorber is being used.

- All connections should be secured by 'push and twist' method.

7. Check the ventilator and its connections.
   - Ensure the ventilator tubing is correctly configured and securely attached.
   - Set the controls for use and ensure an adequate pressure is generated during the inspiratory phase.
   - Check the pressure relief valve and the disconnection alarm function correctly.

8. Ensure the availability of an alternative means (Resuscitation bag and mask/Breathing circuit) to ventilate the lungs.

9. Check the anaesthetic gas-scavenging system
   - Whether it is switched on, if present and is functioning correctly.
   - Ensure that the tubing is attached to the appropriate (expiratory) ports of the breathing system or ventilator.

10. Check all ancillary equipment such as laryngoscopes, intubation aids, intubation forceps, bougies, appropriately sized face masks, airways, tracheal tubes and connectors, etc. are available. Check that the suction apparatus is functioning and that all connections are secure.

11. Ensure that the appropriate monitoring equipment is present, switched on and calibrated ready for use. Set all default alarms as appropriate.

12. Check that the operating table can be moved up and down, tilted laterally and into Trendelenburg/anti-Trendelenburg positions.

For the Subsequent Cases on the OT List

1. Check that the adequate supply of oxygen is available from a reserve oxygen cylinder.
2. Ensure that each vapouriser is adequately filled but not over-filled. A leak test should be performed immediately after changing any vapouriser.
3. Check the breathing system. All connections should be secured by 'push and twist' method. The correct operation of unidirectional valves should be checked if soda lime of circle absorber has been changed.
4. Check the ventilator and its connections. Ensure the availability of an alternative means (Resuscitation bag and mask/Breathing circuit) to ventilate the lungs.
5. Check all ancillary equipment such as laryngo-scopes, intubation aids, intubation forceps, bougies, appropriately sized face masks, airways, tracheal tubes and connectors, etc. are available. Check that the suction apparatus is functioning and that all connections are secure (Figs 1.1 to 1.3).

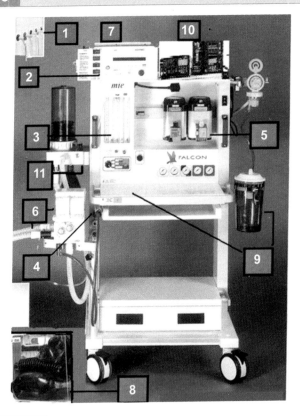

Figure 1.1

(1) Check gas supply connections, pressures and reserve oxygen cylinder, (2) Oxygen analyser, (3) Check the operation of flow meters and oxygen failure device, (4) Check the operation of the emergency oxygen flush and position of bypass control, (5) Check the vapourisers, (6) Check the breathing system, (7) Check the ventilator, (8) Resuscitation bag and mask, (9) Check all Ancillary equipment, (10) Ensure monitoring equipment, (11) Check the anaesthetic gas-scavenging system if present

All connections should be secured by 'push and twist'

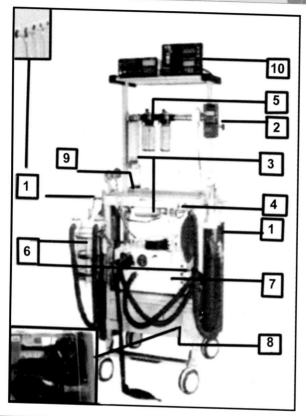

Figure 1.2

(1) Check gas supply connections, pressures and reserve oxygen cylinder, (2) Oxygen analyser, (3) Check the operation of flow meters and oxygen failure devices, (4) Check the operation of the emergency oxygen flush and position of bypass control, (5) Check the vapourisers, (6) Check the breathing system, (7) Check the ventilator, (8) Resuscitation bag and mask, (9) Check all ancillary equipment, (10) Ensure monitoring equipment

All connections should be secured by 'push and twist'

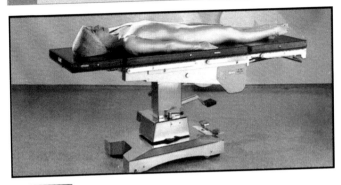

Figure 1.3

Check the operation table for tilt facility prior to administration of spinal anaesthesia

6. Ensure that the appropriate monitoring equipment is present, switched on and calibrated ready for use. Set all default alarms as appropriate.

(Modified from Association of Anaesthetists guidelines, 1997)

Chapter 2

Monitoring Standards

STANDARDS FOR BASIC INTRAOPERATIVE MONITORING

Standard I

Qualified anaesthesia personnel shall be present in the operating room throughout the conduct of all general anaesthetics, regional anaesthetics, and monitored anaesthesia care.

Standard II

During all anaesthetics, the patient's oxygenation, ventilation, circulation and temperature shall be continually evaluated.

Monitoring Methods

Oxygenation

1. *Inspired gas monitoring*: While administering general anaesthesia using an anaesthesia machine, the concentration of oxygen in the patient breathing system shall be monitored by an oxygen analyser. Low oxygen concentration audio/visual/audio-visual alarm should be in use.
2. *Blood oxygenation*: During all anaesthetics, a quantitative method of assessing oxygenation such as a pulse oximetry shall be employed.
   Adequate illumination and exposure of the patient are necessary to assess colour.

Ventilation

1. Every patient receiving general anaesthesia shall have the adequacy of ventilation monitored and continually evaluated.
   - Clinical signs such as chest excursion, observation of the reservoir breathing bag, and auscultation of breath sound may be adequate
   - Monitoring of the CO_2 content and/or volume of expired gas is encouraged.
2. When an endotracheal tube is inserted, its correct positioning in the trachea must be verified by clinical assessment and by identification of carbon dioxide in the expired gas. End-tidal CO_2 analysis, in use from the time of endotracheal tube placement, is encouraged.
3. When a mechanical ventilator is in use, there should be continuous use of a device with audiovisual alarm for detection of disconnection of components of the breathing system.
4. During regional anaesthesia and monitored anaesthesia care, the adequacy of ventilation shall be continuously evaluated, at least by clinical signs.

Circulation

1. *EKG*: All patients receiving anaesthesia shall have their electrocardiogram monitored continuously.
2. *Arterial blood pressure:* All patients receiving anaesthesia shall have arterial blood pressure and

heart rate determined and evaluated at least every five minutes and recorded.

3. *Pulse plethysmography or oximetry*: Every patient receiving anaesthesia shall have, in addition to the above, circulatory function continually evaluated by at least one of the following methods: palpation of a pulse, auscultation of heart sounds, monitoring of a tracing of intra-arterial pressure, ultrasound peripheral pulse monitoring, pulse plethysmography or oximetry.

Body Temperature

Facility (thermometer or electronic thermister) for temperature monitoring shall be there all the times while administering anaesthesia. When changes in body temperature are intended, anticipated or suspected, the temperature shall be measured/monitored continuously.

SPECIAL INTRAOPERATIVE MONITORING

Invasive Arterial Blood Pressure Monitoring

Intra-arterial blood pressure should be monitored in following situations:

- Excessive bleeding.
- Difficulty in recording NIBP, such as morbid obesity, oedema.
- Pregnant females undergoing neurosurgical procedures.

Central Venous Pressure Monitoring (CVP)

CVP should be monitored in parturient having excessive blood loss and massive transfusions and cardiac lesions.

Pulmonary Capillary Wedge Pressure Monitoring (PCWP)

Occasionally required in patients who need accurate titration of fluid management, e.g. in cardiomyopathies.

Indian Society of Anaesthesiologists (ISA) accepted the recommended monitoring standards published by World Federation of Societies of Anaesthesiologists (WFSA) as 'International Standard of Monitoring" in January'1996. Later in 2000, ISA revised guidelines for Indian institutions and hospitals [Adapted from Anaesthesia Monitoring Standards Recommended for India. Ind J Anaesth. 2000; (44): 59], which are as follows:

Pre-Requisites

Professional Status

Only qualified Anaesthesiologists are permitted to administer anaesthesia.

Facilities and Equipment

Resuscitation equipment conforming to national standards must be available at the work place in adequate quantity/quality.

Professional Organisation

Appropriate 'Anaesthesia forums' may be established and will form links with the needed a Authority for training, certification and accreditation.

Records and Statistics

A record of details and course of each anaesthesia procedure should be made and preserved along with the patient's medical record.

Personnel and Workload

Sufficient number of trained anaesthesiologists should be available.

BASIC STANDARDS OF MONITORING

i. Pre-anaesthetic evaluation and adherence to a protocol is mandatory. Service should be administered by qualified anaesthesiologist.

ii. Availability of resuscitation equipment, uninterrupted supply of oxygen and minimum anaesthesia equipment should be confirmed before starting the procedure.

iii. Clinical monitoring of color and pulse should be done every 5 minutes during conduct of anaesthesia.

iv. A light source should be available always.

v. Stethoscope, BP apparatus and thermometer should be available. Basal recording should be made before the start of procedure.

vi. Cardioscope with defibrillator capable of displaying the rate and wave pattern should be available.

DESIRABLE STANDARDS
(Essential Standards for Higher Surgical Workplaces)

1. All basic standards detailed above should be met with.
2. Anaesthetic machine and equipment used should have failure warning facility as well as a checklist for failure correction. Every operating theatre should have at least one operable anaesthetic machine.
3. Periodically calibrated vapouriser (drug specific) should be available.
4. Every procedure should be monitored with Pulse Oxymeter to observe oxygen saturation.
5. Major procedures should be extensively monitored using different equipment such as Airway Pressure Alarm, Oxygen Concentration Analyser, Neuro-Muscular Monitor, Respiratory Volume Monitor, Non-invasive BP Monitor, Capnometer, etc.

Chapter 3

Maternal Physiology in Pregnancy

CHANGES IN MATERIAL PHYSIOLOGY IN PREGNANCY

System	Variable	Change
Respiratory	FRC	-20%
	Vital capacity	No change
	Closing volume	No change
	Minute ventilation	+50%
	Tidal volume	+40%
	Respiratory rate	+15%
	Dead space	No change
	Lung compliance	No change
	Chest wall compliance	-45%
	Airway resistance	-36%
	FEV_1	No change
	Oxygen consumption	+20%
Cardiac	Cardiac output	+43%
	Heart rate	+17%
	Stroke volume	+18%
	SVR	-21%
	PVR	-34%
CNS	Anaesthetic requirement for inhaled anaesthetic agent	-25% to - 40%
	Anaesthetic requirement for spinal anaesthesia	-30%

Contd...

Contd...

System	Variable	Change
GIT	Gastric emptying (during pregnancy)	No change
	Gastric emptying (during labour)	Markedly prolonged
	Gastric acid secretion (during pregnancy)	Decreases
	Lower esophageal sphincter tone	Decreases
Renal	Glomerular filtration rate	Increases
	Blood urea and S creatinine	Decreases
Coagulation profile	Synthesis of various coagulation factors and inhibitory proteins is affected	Hyper-coagulable state

FRC: Functional residual capacity
SVR: Systemic vascular resistance
PVR: Pulmonary vascular resistance

Uterine Blood Flow

At term it is about 10% of cardiac output (600-700 ml/min); in non-pregnant uterus it is 50 ml/min.

Uterine vasculature is maximally dilated due to pregnancy, hence auto-regulation is absent. Blood flow is directly proportional to difference between uterine arterial and venous pressures but inversely proportional to uterine vascular resistance.

Three major factors that decrease uterine blood flow during pregnancy are:

1. Hypotension—due to aortocaval compression, hypovolaemia, regional anaesthesia.
2. Vasoconstriction
   • Due to stress induced endogenous catecholamines release
   • Use of drugs with alpha adrenergic activity.
3. Uterine contractions.

Barbiturates cause a small reduction in uterine blood flow while propofol-midazolam combination can cause slight systemic hypotension; ketamine and etomidate have minimal effects.

Volatile inhalation agents decrease uteroplacental blood flow but in concentration less than 1 MAC their effects are negligible.

Nitrous oxide has minimal effect.

Spinal and epidural anaesthesia do not decrease uterine blood flow *provided* hypotension is avoided.

Placental Transfer of Drugs

Placental transport of anaesthetics occurs primarily by passive diffusion. Factors which promote rapid diffusion are:

• Low molecular weight (< 600 daltons)
• High lipid solubility
• Low degree of ionization
• Low protein binding.

Drugs administered to mother effect the foetus; these effects depend on:

1. Route of administration—IM, IV, epidural or intrathecal.
2. Timing of administration relative to delivery and uterine contractions.
3. Dose of drug.
4. Maturity of foetal organs.
5. Damage to placenta (loss of placental capillary integrity) as seen in hypertension, diabetes and toxaemia, can lead to non-selective transfer of material across placenta.

Currently used anaesthetic drugs have minimal foetal effects despite significant placental transfer.

All inhalation agents, most intravenous agents and opiates cross the placenta.

Muscle relaxants diffuse poorly through the placenta and have minimum effect on foetus because they are highly ionized.

Highly protein bound local anaesthetics diffuse poorly across the placenta (Bupivacaine and Ropivacaine diffuse less than Xylocaine).

Maternally administered ephedrine, betablockers, vasodilators, metoclopramide, phenothiazines are transferred to the foetus.

Atropine and scopalamine crosses the placenta but glycopyrrolate does not do so.

PHYSIOLOGICAL CHANGES OF PREGNANCY AND THEIR ANAESTHETIC IMPLICATIONS

System	Physiological change	Anaesthetic implication
Cardiovascular system	↑ cardiac output (4.5 → 6 L/min) Cardiac output upto 12 L/min in labour	Awareness more likely Important in presence of cardiac disease
	↓ peripheral resistance ↓ blood pressure, especially diastolic	Less hypotensive effect of thiopentone and vasodilators
	↑ organ blood flow, particularly uterus, kidney	Easier venous access
	↑ coagulability of blood	↑ risk of venous thrombosis
	Aortocaval compression in supine position	Lateral tilt required to avoid foetal asphyxia
Respiratory system	↑ minute ventilation (7.5 → 10.5 L/min)	Awareness more likely

Contd....

Contd....

System	Physiological change	Anaesthetic implication
	↓ $PaCO_2$ 40 mm Hg → 30 mm Hg ↓ functional residual capacity ↑ oxygen consumption Congested nasal mucous membranes	↑ ventilation required ↓ oxygen stores, pre-oxygenation necessary Care with nasogastric or nasotracheal tubes
GIT	↓ lower oesophageal sphincter tone ↑ extragastric pressure Delayed gastric emptying	↑ risk of gastric aspiration
Fluid status	↑ blood volume (by 1250 ml) Total body water ↑ by 6-8 litres ↑ red cell volume ↓ plasma concentration of	↑ volume of distribution of drugs; some blood loss tolerated at delivery without requiring replacement

Contd....

Contd....

System	Physiological change	Anaesthetic implication
	sodium, potassium and urea	Recognition of incipient renal failure with normal non-pregnant values
	↓ concentration plasma proteins but ↑ total amount	↑ drug binding
General	Breast enlargement	Difficulty in introducing laryngoscope
	Lumbar lordosis, Ligamental softening	Difficulty in opening up lumbar interspaces, dural tap

Chapter 4

Preoperative and Airway Assessment of Pregnant Patient

The objective of preanaesthetic evaluation is to become familiar with the current surgical illness and co-existing medical conditions, developing a management strategy for perioperative anaesthetic care and establishing a doctor-patient rapport.

The goal is to reduce perioperative morbidity and mortality.

History

This can be facilitated by asking the patients to complete a preoperative questionnaire. Important points to glean from the notes are:

1. Previous illnesses, operations and anaesthetics: Previous exposure to anaesthesia, type of anaesthesia, experience (good/unpleasant), how long ago and complications if any. Complications of previous anaesthesia administrations may be avoided on this occasion. However previous uneventful course does not ensure a repeat performance.

   History of death or major morbidity due to anaesthesia in the family, demands ruling out of conditions such as malignant hyperthermia, scoline apnea and anaphylaxis.

2. Drug therapy: E.g. corticosteroids, insulin, antihypertensive drugs, tranquilizers, digitalis, diuretics, mono-amine oxidase inhibitors, tricyclic antidepressants have important anaesthetic implications.

Drug allergies and drug addiction may be noted.

3. Symptoms referable to the respiratory system: Respiratory reserve, cough, sputum, bronchospasm, ability to expel secretions, Smoking habits, Breathlessness, paroxysmal nocturnal dyspnoea and orthopnoea are important symptoms.

4. Cardiovascular system: Exercise tolerance, Hypertension, Breathlessness, Chest pain. History of hypertension/Pregnancy induced hypertension is particularly important.

   Comfort level while lying in supine position will reveal if the patient is prone to aorto-caval compression/supine hypotension.

5. Tendency to postanaesthetic vomiting: This will affect the choice of anaesthetic drugs.

6. Bleeding tendencies

7. Smoking and alcohol intake: Both are harmful to the mother and child.

   Smokers exhibit a variety of pulmonary disorders, e.g. airway obstruction and reduced lung compliance, diminished peak flow rate, increase in functional residual capacity, diminished diffusing capacity and reduced surfactant.

   It should be stopped 4-6 weeks before surgery to reduce airway hyperreactivity and perioperative pulmonary complications.

   Stopping smoking for 12-24 hours before surgery benefits the cardiovascular system by withdrawing carbon monoxide and nicotine; stopping for a few days will benefit ciliary activity; stopping for 1-2 weeks will reduce sputum volume.

In abdominal operations postoperative chest complications are six times more frequent in smokers than in nonsmokers.

The alcoholic patient may suffer from cirrhosis of the liver, cardiomyopathy, diminished adrenocortical response to stress, electrolyte imbalance, hypoglycaemia, neuropathy and psychosis.

General Physical Examination

Physical examination must be thorough with emphasis on airway, heart, lungs, neurological examination, oral cavity, neck and the back (for spinal).

General Examination

a. Record the height and weight which is important in estimating drug dosages and fluid requirement.
b. Look for cyanosis, jaundice, pigmentation or pallor, oedema over feet and sacral region.
c. The state of nutrition, malnutrition or obesity is noted.

   Weight check for obesity and try to differentiate between fluid retention and true obesity. If Body Mass Index (BMI) is more than of 27, parturients are considered obese.
d. Temperature is recorded.
e. Veins: The state of the veins is noted.

f. A note of blood pressure and resting pulse rate is made. Patient with resting tachycardia is prone to supine hypotension after spinal block.

Blood pressure in supine and left lateral position is taken in a pregnant patient; a drop of more than 15 mm Hg arterial pressure in supine position indicates that the patient is prone to supine hypotension.

g. Respiration is observed for rate, depth and "pattern" while at rest.

h. Psychological state: Is the patient calm, apprehensive, unstable or anxious?

Assessment of Pulmonary Function

Stress is on clinical and monitored signs of respiratory disease, respiratory pattern and character, presence of added sounds on auscultation, localising signs, mediastinal shift, finger clubbing and cyanosis.

Assessment of the Cardiovascular System

The aim is to look for evidence of coronary artery disease, valvular lesions, arrhythmias and to assess the cardiac reserve. Serious heart disease can be asymptomatic. Acute myocardial infarction can be present without obvious symptoms.

Nervous System

Examination of the nervous system including the spine particularly where spinal or epidural block is envisaged, is done.

PRE-ANAESTHETIC CHECK SHEET

Date ....

Name ....

Weight ....

Height..

Surgeon ....

Operation ....

Have you had an anaesthetic before?

Have you or your relatives had a complication from an anaesthetic?

Have you got any crowns or caps on your front teeth? Have you got any loose teeth?

Do you wear contact lenses?

Are you allergic to any drugs? If so, which ones?

Do you have allergic asthma or skin rashes?

Do you smoke? How many?

Do you get short of breath after climbing stairs?

Have you had:
   High blood pressure
   Pain in the chest
   Heart disease
   Epilepsy
   Bleeding problems
   Diabetes
   Asthma
   Bronchitis
   Jaundice

Any other medical condition you suffer from?

Are you "on the pill"? ⎤
                        ⎥ (for women only)
Are you pregnant? ⎦

Are you on any medicines? If so, which ones, and how often?

Is there anything else the anaesthetist needs to know about you?

If the answer to any of these questions is yes, please give a few details

Assessment of the Airway

Maintenance of an adequate airway at all times is one of the prime duties of an anaesthesiologist. Endotracheal intubation must be smooth and quick; to achieve this end, preoperative airway evaluation is done; it requires no equipment, is entirely non-invasive and takes less than a minute to perform.

1. The examination first focuses on the teeth; if the upper incisors are big or the maxillary teeth are anterior to mandibular teeth then there is difficulty in inserting the laryngoscope blade in the oral cavity. Poor dentition increases the risk of dental damage and dislodgement during airway manipulation.

   Loose teeth must be identified preoperatively and protected with a dental guard or occasionally removed.

2. If the patient is able to protrude the mandible beyond the maxilla, this signifies good temporomandibular joint function and good mouth opening resulting in easy insertion of the laryngoscope.

3. If the distance between the upper and lower incisors on opening the mouth is more than 3 cm, then laryngoscopy is easy.

4. A large tongue or a narrow, highly arched palate reduces the oropharyngeal volume and make the laryngoscopy and visualisation of the glottis difficult.

5. If the distance between the notch of thyroid cartilage and symphysis mentii with the neck fully extended, is more than 5 cm, intubation is easy.

6. A short, thick neck and restricted movement of head and neck make intubation difficult. Patients should be able to touch their chin to their chest and also be able to extend their neck as far posteriorly as possible.

If endotracheal intubation is anticipated to be difficult, then the anaesthesiologist has the time to plan and take suitable measures to overcome the problem.

Additional Bedside Tests

1. Exercise tolerance.
2. The breath-holding test. The resting patient takes a full inspiration and holds breath. A time of 25 sec or longer may be taken as normal. A time of 15 sec or less indicates diminished cardiorespiratory reserve.
3. The forced expiratory volume and vital capacity can be readily measured by pocket-sized Micro-spirometers.
4. The Wright peak flow-meter can be used to measure peak expiratory flow rate.
5. Pulse oximetry.

Investigations

Haemoglobin, haematocrit, total and differential blood counts and complete urine analysis are a part of every preoperative work-up. Symptoms suggestive of hepatic, renal or metabolic disease are thoroughly investigated by laboratory studies specific for the system concerned.

- Haemoglobin level should be measured in all pregnant patients.
- Bleeding time is an unreliable test; a normal bleeding time gives false safety. Prolonged bleeding time needs to be investigated further.
- Clotting time (CT) may be normal even in presence of gross deficiencies (Visible clot requires only a little amount of plasma factor 4).
- Platelet count is an important investigation in parturients as it may be low in Pre-Eclamptic Toxaemia (PET) and HELLP syndrome.
- PT and PTTK may be prolonged. It indicates underlying HELLP syndrome, severe PET, Liver disease or DIC.
- Blood grouping is essential to rule out Rh-incompatibility of newborn and for blood transfusion in cases of bleeding.

Special Investigations

Special investigations may be required if the parturient has some medical disorders, e.g. valvular cardiac disease needs further cardiac evaluation like electrocardiography and echocardigraphy.

Radiation exposure should be avoided during pregnancy, but it can be done if medical problem overweighs the risk of exposure.

All extensive surgery should be preceded by a baseline electrolyte panel as a basis for postoperative fluid and electrolyte replacement therapy. Serum sodium, potassium and calcium levels are important.

- Ultrasonography of uterus: Position of placenta should be known especially in cases of low lying placenta and previous caesarean section. If there is placenta previa with history of previous caesarean section, the possibility of caesarean hysterectomy must be kept in mind.

Risk Stratification

American Society of Anaesthesiology (ASA) classification of patient's physical status (ASA status) gives broad information of risk involved during surgery and anaesthesia.

ASA status I	Healthy patient.
ASA status II	Mild systemic disease well controlled with no or minimal restricted activity.
ASA status III	Systemic disease, moderate in intensity with constant threat; moderately restricted activity.
ASA status IV	Severe systemic disease, uncontrolled despite therapy; limited activity, constant threat.
ASA status V	Moribund, likely to die with or without surgery.

E is added for emergency surgery.

ASA CLASSIFICATION OF OPERATIONS

Class 1

The patient has no organic, physiological, biochemical or psychiatric disorder. The pathology for which surgery is planned is simple and does not involve a major systemic disturbance (Fibroid uterus in a healthy female).

Class 2

Mild to moderate systemic disturbance or distress caused by the condition to be treated surgically or by other pathological disturbance limiting patient's reserve to overcome stress, e.g. mild heart disease, mild, controlled diabetes or hypertension, obesity and chronic bronchitis.

Class 3

Severe systemic disease or disturbance from whatever cause, although the degree of disability may not be defined with finality, e.g. severely limiting heart disease, diabetes or hypertension with systemic complications, healed myocardial infarction.

Class 4

Severe life threatening disorders which are not correctable by operation, e.g. ruptured aortic aneurysm with profound shock or major cerebral trauma with rapidly increasing intracranial pressure. Such patients require operation as resuscitative effort and may need little or no anaesthesia.

Classification of Operations on Basis of Urgency

Immediate

Resuscitation simultaneous with surgery, e.g. ruptured uterus with bleeding.

Urgent

Caesarean section for foetal distress.

Scheduled

Early surgery but not immediately life saving, e.g. hysterectomy for malignancy.

Elective

Operation at a time which suits to patient and surgeon, e.g. elective hysterectomy.

THE ASSESSMENT OF THE AIRWAY

The prime responsibility of an anaesthesiologist is to maintain an adequate airway for effective gas exchange; the inability to do so is a prominent cause of anaesthetic deaths. The ten most common critical incidents during anaesthesia are related to failure to ventilate (70%), laryngoscope malfunction, premature extubation and problems with endotracheal tube. Difficult or failed intubation is encountered in approximately 5% of obstetric general anaesthesia; the incidence of failed intubation is eight times higher in pregnant patients than in other surgical patients. The causes are weight gain, breast enlargement, airway edema, reduction of functional residual capacity, and delayed gastric emptying time.

Classification of Difficult Airway

The severity of difficulty in maintaining an airway for mask ventilation can range from zero to infinity. Zero degree means that no external effort or internal airway device is needed to maintain a patent airway. An infinite degree means that despite maximal efforts and use of oropharyngeal and nasopharyngeal airways, the ability to maintain patent airway is nearly impossible.

Mallampati Grading (Fig. 4.1)

Assessment is made with the patient sitting upright, with head in neutral position, mouth opened as wide as possible and tongue protuded out maximally. The observer is seated directly in front of the patient. Based on the structures visible on mouth opening, the grading is made.

Class I: Soft palate, fauces, uvula, tonsillar pillars can be seen.

Class II: All the above can be seen except the tonsillar pillars.

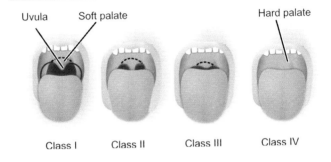

Figure 4.1

Mallampati grading of airway

Class III: Only soft palate and base of uvula seen.

Class IV: Not even the uvula can be visualised.

CORMACK AND LEHANE CLASSIFICATION

Four grades are recognised based on the view obtained on direct laryngoscopy, using a Macintosh laryngoscope blade (Fig. 4.2).

Grade I: Full view of the glottis.

Grade II: Only posterior commissure visible.

Grade III: Only tip of the epiglottis visible.

Grade IV: No glottic structure visible.

Grade I = intubation is easy; Grade IV= intubation is difficult.

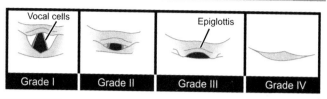

Figure 4.2

Cormack and Lehane classification

Airway Assessment and Management of Difficult Airways

A careful, pre-anaesthetic evaluation should identify the vast majority of difficult airways.

The evaluation should include an assessment of:

1. Length of upper incisors— if long, difficult to put in a laryngoscope.
2. Maxillary teeth anterior to Mandibular teeth— difficult laryngoscopy.
3. Protrusion of mandibular teeth anterior to maxillary teeth, possible—good temporomandibular joint function, good mouth opening, easy laryngoscopy.
4. Inter-incisor distance >3 cm—laryngoscope easily inserted into mouth.
5. Size of tongue in relation to oral cavity— large size represents difficulty.
6. Narrowness of palate—should not appear very narrow or highly arched.
7. Thyro-mental distance more than 7 cm—larynx easy to visualise.
8. Length and thickness of neck—thick, short neck represents difficulty.

9   Range of motion of head and neck—restricted
    movements cause difficulty (neck extension <35
    degrees).

MANAGEMENT OF DIFFICULT AIRWAY

Techniques for difficult intubation:
> Alternative laryngoscope blades
> Awake intubation
> Blind intubation oral /nasal
> Fibreoptic intubation
> Intubating stylet
> Light wand
> Retrograde intubation
> Surgical airway

Techniques for difficult ventilation:
> Oesophageal-tracheal combitube
> Intratracheal jet stylet
> Laryngeal mask
> Airways oral/nasopharyngeal
> Rigid ventilating bronchoscope
> Surgical airway access
> Transtracheal jet ventilation
> Two person mask ventilation

Risk factors for intubation and hypoxia specific to the pregnant woman.

1. Pharyngo-Laryngeal oedema
2. Weight gain.
3. Increased breast size.
4. Full dentition.
5. Rapid onset of hypoxaemia during apnoea as a result of decreased functional residual capacity, decreased

cardiac output due to aortocaval compression and increased oxygen consumption.

Prophylaxis

1. Regional versus general anaesthesia: The recent decline in maternal mortality can be attributed to increased use of regional anaesthesia in obstetrics.
2. Preparation for general anaesthesia:
   a. Optimal positioning of the patient for intubation.
   b. Preoxygenation for 3 minutes or 4 deep breaths with 100% O_2.
   c. Aspiration prophylaxis.

The patient who cannot be intubated but can be ventilated by mask: The options are:
1. Awaken the patient.
2. Use of tracheostomy or cricothyroidotomy.
3. Continue anaesthesia with mask ventilation while assistant maintains cricoid pressure—the failed intubation drill.

The sequence of events in this drill are as follows (Fig. 4.3):
1. Maintain cricoid pressure
2. Place patient in complete left lateral position and ventilate with mask; Avoid left lateral position if ventilation is difficult in this position.
3. Maintain oxygenation by intermittent positive pressure ventilation with 100% O_2
4. For persistent airway obstruction, release cricoid pressure gradually, if patient is in complete left

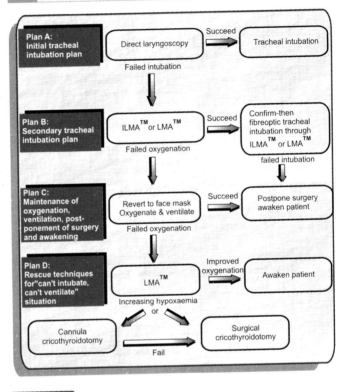

Figure 4.3

Difficult airway protocol

lateral position with head down and breathing spontaneously.

5. If ventilation and oxygenation are easy, nitrous oxide and a potent halogenated agent can be added to allow establishment of surgical anaesthesia via face mask ventilation with spontaneous breathing.

6. Pass 33-36 Fr. gastric tube via the mouth and aspirate the gastric contents and instill a non-particulate antacid. Withdraw the tube and suction the oropharynx during the withdrawal.

7. Level the table and place patient supine and allow the operation to continue using inhalational anaesthesia with a face mask (Paediatrician should be present at the time of delivery).

The patient who cannot be intubated or cannot be ventilated by face mask. When cannot ventilate cannot intubate (CVCI) situation develops, options are (Fig. 4.4):

1. Use of laryngeal mask airway (LMA).
2. Use of combitube.
3. Transtracheal jet ventilation (TTJV).
4. Cricothyroidotomy/tracheostomy.

Both the LMA and the combitube work well in CVCI situation.

- Both are likely to work as ventilatory mechanisms.
- Both can be inserted blindly, quickly, and a low level of skill is required.
- Very few complications seen.
- More chances of complications with TTJV, e.g. barotrauma.

Disadvantages

Both are supraglottic ventilatory mechanisms (combitube enters the oesophagus 99% of the times). They cannot solve a truly glottic or subglottic problem such as glottic spasm, oedema, tumour, abscess.

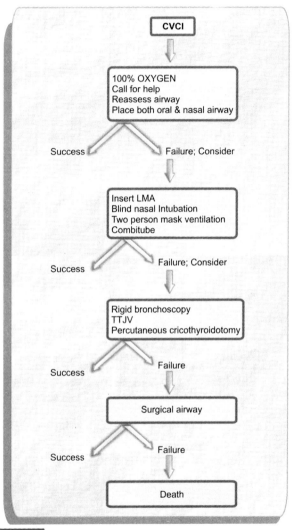

Figure 4.4

Algorithm for cannot ventilate, cannot intubate (CVCI)

With a truly glottic or subglottic problem, the solution is to get below the site of lesion by TTJV or ETT or surgical airway.

Extubation

For patients with difficult airway, extubation should be done when patient is fully awake and breathing is adequate.

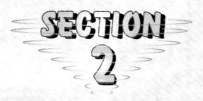

SECTION 2

ANAESTHESIA AND PREGNANCY

Chapter 5

Non-Obstetric Surgery in Pregnancy

ANAESTHESIA FOR THE PREGNANT PATIENT UNDERGOING NON-OBSTETRIC SURGERY

Surgery during pregnancy is necessary in about .5-2% of pregnancies. The difficulty arises when surgery has to be performed during the period of organogenesis (13th to 56th day after conception) or when foetal viability may be compromised.

Most common procedures are Cerclage procedure, Acute abdomen, Maternal trauma and Correction of decompensating cardiac lesion. Major procedures such as craniotomy and cardiopulmonary bypass have also been performed in the pregnant patient with good outcomes for mother and foetus.

GOALS IN ANAESTHETIC MANAGEMENT

1. Maternal safety
   - Good preoperative preparation and evaluation
   - Optimum anaesthetic management
   - Adequate analgesia during and after surgery but without foetal depression
2. Foetal safety
   - Prevention of pre-term labour
   - Avoidance of teratogenic drugs.
   - Optimum uteroplacental perfusion to prevent foetal asphyxiation and hypoxia.

Anaesthetic management now involves two patients: mother and foetus. Alterations in maternal physiology involve every organ system but those most important to anaesthetic management include the following:

Respiratory

Higher oxygen consumption, lower functional residual capacity, lower CO_2 levels due to elevated minute ventilation, greater incidence of difficult intubations are the problems faced.

The pregnant patient is more prone to hypoxia. Administer oxygen and monitor oxygen saturation by pulse oximetry.

Normocarbia should be maintained during controlled ventilation because low CO_2 levels will compromise uteroplacental perfusion.

Postoperative pain will cause rapid shallow respiration which will further decrease CO_2 levels, hence the need for good analgesia but without foetal depression.

Cardiovascular

Increased blood volume and cardiac output, dilutional anaemia, aortocaval compression in supine position and hypercoaguable state of blood is seen during pregnancy.

Any gravida with a coexisting heart disease has an increased risk of cardiac decompensation, especially those with mitral valve involvement. It needs aggressive medical treatment; if it fails, surgical correction is needed.

Gastrointestinal

Gastric volume and pH may not be altered till third trimester of pregnancy but gastroesophageal sphincter tone is usually reduced; hence the need to prevent regurgitation and aspiration of gastric content during surgery. Give H_2 blockers preoperatively.

Central Nervous System

MAC for inhalation agents and local anaesthetic requirements are both decreased during pregnancy.

Teratogenic effects of anaesthetics have never been conclusively shown.

The drugs of most concern are nitrous oxide and the benzodiazepines.

No adverse effects of nitrous oxide have been demonstrated in human pregnancy.

The benzodiazepines have been associated with cleft lip anomalies.

The inhalation agents, narcotics, intravenous agents, local anaesthetics are safe during pregnancy.

Maintenance of maternal oxygenation and uterine perfusion preserves foetal oxygenation. Maintain maternal cardiac output, oxygen saturation and uterine blood flow; avoid maternal hypoxia and hypotension at all cost.

Prevention and treatment of preterm labour are the most difficult problems to overcome perioperatively; preterm delivery is the most common cause of foetal loss. It is probably not related to anaesthetic management but to the underlying disease and the surgical procedure.

Tocolytic agents (Beta sympathomimetic drugs) are used before 32 weeks' gestation and are effective for 24 to 48 hours only. They cause tachycardia, hypotension and cardiac arrhythmias.

If Magnesium sulphate is used, it interacts with muscle relaxants and also causes CNS depression. In the neonate it can cause some alteration of neuromuscular function.

Abdominal laparoscopic procedures during pregnancy present additional risks to the foetus. Pneumoperitoneum pressures are kept between 8 and 12 mm Hg because above this range uterine blood flow is severely compromised. The placement of trocars and other instruments can injure the uterus.

RECOMMENDED GUIDELINES IN THE MANAGEMENT OF THE PREGNANT PATIENT FOR NONOBSTETRIC SURGERY

Timing of Surgery

- As far as possible, delay the proposed operative procedure till the second or third trimester. The foetus is most vulnerable with regard to teratogenic effects until the 12th week of pregnancy.
- The risk of spontaneous abortion remains high even in the second trimester.

Choice of Drugs

- Use anaesthetic agents with a known history of foetal safety. Understandably, this is a must during the first trimester, but must also be observed beyond the stage of organogenesis.
- Use drugs and techniques that preserve utero-placental perfusion and prevent uterine irritability or premature contractions.

Promote Foetal Well-being

- Keep all maternal physiological functions at an optimum.
- Ensure good uteroplacental perfusion by
  a. Maintaining normal maternal systemic arterial blood pressure.
  b. Promoting maternal normocarbia and normal acid-base balance.
  c. Preventing uterine irritability and hypertonicity.
  d. Using drugs to achieve the desired therapeutic end points while avoiding foetal toxicity and depression.
- Perform intensive foetal monitoring especially during surgery and in the immediate postoperative period.

Promote Maternal Well-being

- Provide optimal emotional and psychological support, particularly during the preoperative preparation of the patient.

- Allay anxiety and promote a stress-free environment perioperatively.
- Perform intensive monitoring during surgery.
- Ensure optimal postoperative pain control.
- Encourage multidisciplinary care of the pregnant patient, particularly if medical problems are present. Involve the relevant specialty service to ensure that the non-obstetric problems of the mother are well managed.

PRINCIPLES FOR ANAESTHETIC MANAGEMENT OF THE PARTURIENT < 20 WEEKS GESTATION

- Postpone surgery until second trimester, if possible.
- Request preoperative assessment by an obstetrician.
- Counsel the patient preoperatively.
- Use a nonparticulate antacid as aspiration prophylaxis.
- Monitor and maintain oxygenation, normocarbia, normotension, and euglycaemia.
- Use regional anaesthesia when appropriate.
- Avoid N_2O in high concentrations during general anaesthesia.
- Document foetal heart tones before and after the procedure.

Laparoscopic Surgery in Pregnancy

It requires general anaesthesia and carbon dioxide is insufflated into the peritoneal cavity.

Abdominal laparoscopic procedures during pregnancy can present additional risks to the fetus. Carbon dioxide insufflation can decrease uteroplacental perfusion and cause foetal acidosis.

Pneumoperitoneal pressures should be in the range of 8 to 12 mm Hg because above this range, the uterine blood flow may be severely compromised because of increased intra-abdominal pressure.

Placement of trocars and other instruments may injure the gravid uterus.

Chapter 6

Anaesthesia for Assisted Reproductive Techniques

Although Assisted Reproductive Techniques (ART) include many techniques, the basic pattern remains the same constituted by hormonal stimulation, oocyte retrieval, *in vitro* fertilization and transfer to the fallopian tube or uterine cavity.

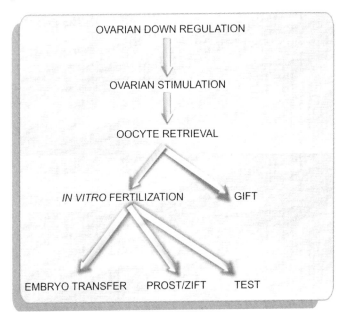

GIFT —gamete intrafallopian transfer
PROST—pronuclear stage tubal transfer
ZIFT—zygote intrafallopian tube transfer
TEST—tubal embryo intrafallopian tube transfer

ART PATHWAY

Impact of anaesthesia on embryogenesis is still unexplored to a large extent. Potential anaesthetic interactions may include direct or indirect effect of the anaesthetic state or agents on gamete and embryo development. Cause-effect relationships are difficult to establish.

- Local anaesthetics appear to have minimal impact on ART outcome. Drugs administered during induction of general anaesthesia have been found in follicles
- Thiopentone 5 mg/kg and Propofol 2.5 mg/kg has been used without any detrimental effect on fertilizations or embryo development.
- Midazolam and fentanyl may be used for premedication. Midazolam appeared to accelerate embryo development (probably increases DNA replication).
- Addition of Propofol did not have negative impact on embryos, implantation rates and probability of clinical pregnancy.
- Nitrous Oxide remains an enigma; it inhibits Methionine synthetase activity and DNA synthesis, it was speculated to affect fertilization and cleavage of human oocytes. Although, in human studies it is found to be safe, but its use in oocyte retrieval should be avoided.
- Halothane when compared with Isoflurane in IVF, has been noted to lower significantly the pregnancy and birth rates (halothane increases the number of abnormal mitoses).

Anaesthesia for Oocyte Retrieval

It is usually done transvaginally but sometimes transabdominal also. Local infiltration with 1% Lidocaine gives poor results with impaired oocyte recovery rates and frequent conversion to GA, thus should be avoided.

- Ketamine 1 mg/kg and Midazolam 0.15 mg/kg are sufficient to retrieve oocyte transvaginally.
- Spinal, epidural with bupivacaine and endotracheal general anaesthesia have been used without any untoward event. Spinal may be preferred over epidural because of less amount of drug used and minimal failure and turnover rate.
- Spinal anaesthesia with Lidocaine 1.5% hyperbaric (45 mg) with Fentanyl 10 mcg, provides excellent anaesthesia with minimal doses of drugs used and short recovery profile.
- GA can be used and the preferred technique is TIVA with Propofol (titrated dose) Fentanyl 50-100 mcg, with Midazolam 1-2 mg as an optional premedicant. Most patients can be managed maintaining spontaneous ventilation with high flow oxygen mask. Isoflurane is the preferred inhalation agent if need arises.

Embryo Transfer

Embryo transfer is relatively painless. Rarely sensitive and anxious female may require intravenous analgesia and sedation.

PROST, ZIFT, TEST and GIFT

Done by laparoscopy; can be done under local, regional or general anaesthesia (GA). GA often provide optimal immobile conditions for placing the embryo in the fallopian tubes.

Post-Anaesthesia Care

- Postoperative pain is treated with fentanyl 25-50 mcg IV.
- NSAIDs are avoided because they can effect embryo implantation.
- Metoclopramide and Droperidol can be used as antiemetics.
- Patients must be hemodynamically stable, able to take and retain oral fluids, ambulate and void prior to discharge.

Chapter 7

Anaesthesia for Foetal Surgery

Intrauterine Foetal Surgery

With advancing medical technology and knowledge it is now possible to tackle some congenital lesions of foetus in the womb of mother at an early stage before it can have its adverse sequelae. The foetus tolerates surgery well and heals rapidly with little or no scarring. It is established now that the foetus can feel the pain and react adversely to it.

Important Issues

1. Maternal safety
2. Avoidance of foetal asphyxia
3. Avoidance of teratogenic drugs
4. Adequate foetal anaesthesia, foetal monitoring
5. Uterine relaxation
6. Prevention of preterm labour.

Principles of Management

- Communication with the surgeon to determine the surgical approach and need for uterine relaxation to plan the anaesthetic technique.
- Many of the anaesthetic considerations for foetal procedures and surgery are identical to those for non-obstetric surgery during pregnancy.

Foetal procedures can be divided into 2 subgroups on the basis of anaesthetic requirements:

Placental or cord procedures	*Direct foetal procedures*
Procedures that only require a needle insertion into the uterus but not into the foetus, such as intrauterine infusions, laser surgical photo-coagulation of the communicating placental circulation for twin-twin transfusion syndrome (TTTS) and radio-frequency umbilical cord ablation for managing twin reversed arterial perfusion (TRAP).	Procedures performed directly on the fetus and the Ex-utero Intrapartum Treatment (EXIT) proce-dure. Common indica-tions for surgery on the foetus are conditions if not corrected early will lead to malformed neonate such as obstruc-tion in urinary tracts with hydronephrosis, lung cysts, diaphragmatic hernia, congenital cardiac defects, etc.

SPECIAL CONSIDERATION FOR FOETAL SURGERY

- The foetus must be monitored and anaesthetized.
- Premature labour must be prevented.
- Avoid factors that decrease uterine blood flow resulting in foetal acidosis.
- Maintain FHR because foetal cardiac output is mainly dependant on foetal heart rate.

- Anaesthesia in mother with Halothane or Isoflurane at 1 MAC or less is safe for foetus.

Maternal Considerations and their Effect on Foetus

- Though mother is not the primary patient, factors affecting the mother have an effect on the foetus.
- Uterine incision can stimulate uterine tone and affect placental circulation (reduced blood flow).
- Increased uterine activity, foetal manipulation, direct compression of vessels, anaesthetics, maternal hypotension, hyperventilation and hypocarbia can alter uterine and umbilical blood flow.

Monitoring the Foetus

Objective: To detect foetal hypoxia, asphyxia and distress at an early stage.

- Foetal heart rate (FHR),
- Pulse oximetry,
- Ultrasonography,
- Blood gases and pH,
- Foetal EEG, ECG, continuous monitoring of blood gases, tissue pH and blood flow can also be monitored.

Prevention of Pre-Term Labour

Tocolytic agents used for prevention of pre-term labour are:

- Preoperative—Indomethacin

- Intraoperative—Isoflurane, Magnesium sulfate, Nitroglycerine
- Postoperative—Magnesium sulfate, Nitroglycerine, Beta-adrenergic agents.

Anaesthesia Techniques

General anaesthesia (GA) should be preferred over regional anaesthesia.

GA offers immobility and anaesthesia of foetus, maintenance of normal maternal-foetal perfusion and, muscle relaxation, uterine relaxation, analgesia and amnesia to mother.

- These patients are very anxious, and must be counseled about invasive monitors, preoperative tocolytics, epidural catheters for postoperative analgesia, etc.
- They must have adequate cardiopulmonary reserve to tolerate blood loss (which is significant) and prolonged and intense tocolytic therapy.
- For transfusion of the foetus, O-negative cytomegalovirus-negative, irradiated blood is used.
  1. NPO as usual, Midazolam if needed preoperative as premedicant.
  2. A technique using halogenated agent (Isoflurane) to provide maternal and foetal anaesthesia as well as uterine relaxation, is used.
  3. Left uterine displacement and rapid induction with sodium pentothal and succinylcholine is done.

4. Maintenance with Isoflurane <1 MAC and 50% oxygen-nitrous oxide mixture.
5. Opioids are given as needed.
6. For the foetus, anaesthesia is provided with fentanyl 25-50 mcg; paralysis by Pancuronium or Rocuronium 3 mg IM. Pancuronium increases the heart rate in foetus, hence preferred.
7. Tocolysis is provided by Nitroglycerine 20 mcg/kg/min which is better than high dose Isoflurane. Additional tocolysis is obtained by Magnesium Sulfate (4 gm/30 minutes followed by 1-2 gm/hour).
8. Mean arterial pressure is maintained at 65 mm Hg.
9. Extubation is done using lidocaine or opioids to minimise straining.
10. Postoperatively premature labour is the most important complication, hence the need for intensive and prolonged tocolytic therapy.

FETOSCOPY

- More procedures are performed using fetoscopy which greatly reduces the risk of postoperative complications because there is less disturbance of the uterus and less tocolysis is needed.
- Vaginal delivery is possible after fetoscopy in contrast to open hysterectomy where an upper uterine incision mandates subsequent caesarean delivery.

— Anaesthetic goals for fetoscopic procedures are the same as for open surgery.
— CO_2 is used to displace the amniotic fluid to allow visualisation of the operative field. This results in hypercarbia and acidosis which is corrected by hyperventilation.
— Helium, Water, Glycine, Hartmann solution have been used to avoid acidosis following use of CO_2.
— High insufflation pressure can lead to decreased placental flow and hypoxia.

SECTION
3

OBSTETRIC ANAESTHESIA
AND ANALGESIA

Chapter 8

Labour Analgesia

Every parturient experiences some pain during child birth; the intensity of labour pain varies from patient to patient. With advent of newer drugs, modalities and strategies, the pain relief during labour is becoming more and more popular. Psychological and physical preparations play an important role in tolerating the labour pains. Other factors such as parity, presentation, anxiety, age and baby's weight also play a contributing role in pain modulation.

Pain during Labour

A painful labour has detrimental effects on both the mother and foetus. Pain causes hyperventilation and sympathetic stimulation resulting in release of catecholamines, with the following effects:

1. Maternal oxygen-haemoglobin dissociation curve shifts to the left during hyperventilation thus reducing foetal oxygenation.
2. There is maternal hypoventilation in between labour pains resulting in less amount of available oxygen for transfer across the placenta. This, combined with decreased uterine blood flow due to catecholamine release, worsens foetal hypoxaemia.
3. Maternal acidosis occurs as a result of lactic acid production from skeletal muscle activity and from free fatty acid production because of sympathetic stimulation. This results in incoordinate uterine action and prolonged labour.

4. Hypertensive response due to sympathetic stimulation is particularly harmful to the mother who is already hypertensive.

Causes of Labour Pain

- Stretching of the cervix during dilatation
- Ischaemia of the muscle wall of the uterus with build up of lactate
- Stretching of the vagina and perineum in the second stage.

Ideal Pain Relief

Should
- Provide good analgesia
- Be safe for the mother and baby
- Be predictable in its effects
- Be reversible if necessary
- Be simple and easy to administer
- Be mother controlled.

Should not
- Interfere with progress of labour
- Interfere with ambulation of mother
- Be associated with adverse effects.

Various methods used for pain relief during labour are as follows:

Non-pharmacological Methods

1. Lamaze's psychoprophylaxis
2. Hypnosis

3. Acupuncture
4. Transcutaneous electric nerve stimulation (TENS).

Pharmacological Methods

Inhalational anaesthetic agents
1. Nitrous oxide
2. Enflurane
3. Isoflurane
4. Desflurane.

Systemic analgesics
1. Opioids
2. Tranquilizers
3. Sedatives
4. Ketamine.

Regional Analgesia

Epidural analgesia
Combined spinal epidural analgesia
Walking epidural.

Common Modalities in Practice

Many of the drugs and techniques used over the years (Chloroform and Trichloroethylene are now obsolete) have been replaced with newer ones which are more effective and safe.

Relaxation and Massage

Anything that helps in relief of parturient's pain, if it does not harm the patient, is acceptable. The removal of anxiety by educating the patient about the physiology of pregnancy and events of labour, various methods of analgesia that are available, training in relaxation techniques, are of great help and are usually taught in antenatal classes.

The Lamaze technique: The mother distracts herself from the pain by concentrating on pictures or other objects in the room and by breathing exercises. Conventional analgesic drugs are allowed in this method.

Transcutaneous eletrical nerve stimulation (TENS): is application of pulsed electrical current through surface electrodes placed on skin. Four electrodes are placed, one on either side of the spine, T10 to L1 for first stage of labour and S2 to S4 for the second stage.

It is thought to work by low frequency stimulation increasing endorphin production and by high frequency stimulation closing the "gate" in the spinal cord to the transmission of pain impulses.

TENS is easy to apply, non-toxic and effective in removing moderate to severe contraction pains of normal labour.

INHALATIONAL ANAESTHETIC AGENTS

Nitrous Oxide

Entonox is premixed 50:50 mixture of nitrous oxide and oxygen which does not interfere with uterine contractions and has no effect on the foetus. Entonox is self-administered through a face mask held by the patient;

the patient cannot take excess amount because the grip on the mask is lost and the mask displaced before consciousness is lost. The mixture improves foetal oxygenation and has a very short half life. Satisfactory analgesia is obtained in about 50% of the patients.

Higher concentrations of nitrous oxide (70%) improve quality of analgesia but produce unconsciousness in a significant number of patients.

During first stage labour, inhalation must begin with the onset of contractions because it takes about 45 seconds for the analgesic effect to be obtained. Deep and slow breathing is encouraged; no inhalation is allowed in between uterine contractions.

In second stage of labour, pains are at regular intervals; it is possible to start inhalation a minute before the pain is expected and to continue until the pain is maximum, followed by bearing down.

Side Effects

- Lightheadedness, drowsiness, confusion, unconsciousness.
- Nausea and vomiting.
- Voluntary hyperventilation to improve analgesia may result in hypocapnia, dizziness and tetany.
- Maternal hyperventilation affects foetal oxygenation adversely.

Enflurane and Isoflurane

Halogenated ethers when used in subanaesthetic concentrations provide good analgesia. They are used via draw-over vapourisers. Because of low solubility coefficient, these inhalational agents have fast inductions and emergence. There is no increase in blood loss or neonatal depression in subanaesthetic concentrations. Both Enflurane (1%) and Isoflurane (.75%) given by intermittent inhalation during first stage of labour produce better analgesia than 50% nitrous oxide but cause more maternal sedation.

Desflurane is another safe and effective inhalation agent for labour analgesia, in subanaesthetic doses but is associated with amnesia. Used as 1% - 4.5% in oxygen, it is very effective but is expensive and requires modified vapouriser for administration.

Sedatives

This includes benzodiazepines which act by binding to benzodiazepine receptors. Diazepam, midazolam and lorazepam are common drugs. Benzodiazepines are unsuitable for labour analgesia because of poor analgesic properties; they are used mainly for their anxiolytic effects.

Systemic Opioids

They provide effective analgesia but with undesirable side effects. Opioids cross the placenta and depress the foetus; hence used only in early labour. In the mother they cause nausea, vomiting, drowsiness and disorientation. Morphine has a more potent depressant effect on the neonate, hence pethidine is more popular.

Continuous infusion or patient controlled administration (PCA) of opioids can provide useful analgesia when regional blocks are contraindicated.

Pethidine 10–25 mg IV or 25–50 mg IM (maximum dose 100 mg) is used in early labour, where delivery is not expected for at least 4 hours.

Promethazine 25-50 mg IM alone or combined with Pethidine, reduces anxiety, nausea and opioid requirement without much effect on foetus.

Fentanyl 50-100 mcg/hour IV has also been used.

Systemic Opioids

Drugs	Dose	Peak (hours)	Duration (hours)	Precautions
Morphine	10 mg IM	1–2	2.5–4	Impaired ventilation
	2.5 mg IV	0.3	1.5–2	Asthma, Liver failure, ↑ICT
Pethidine	50-75 mg IM	0.5–1	3–4	Accumulation of metabolites can cause seizures;
	20-50 mg IV		2–3	Interact with MAO inhibitors
Fentanyl	50-100 mcg IM		1–2	Cumulative effect
	25-50 mcg IV		0.5–1	
Remifentanil	1 mcg/kg bolus infusion at .1–.2 mcg/kg/min			Very short acting potent drug
Pentazocine	40-60 mg IM	0.5-1		May cause psychomimetic effects
	20-40 mg IV			
Butorphanol	2 mg IM	0.5-1	4–6	Psychomimetic effects;
	1 mg IV		3–4	maternal sedation

Ketamine

Ketamine alone or in combination has been used to provide pain relief during labour. It is most useful when given just before delivery or as adjuvant to regional anaesthesia.

Used as a continuous infusion after a bolus of 0.2 mg/kg intravenously, it is found to provide adequate analgesia for 1st stage of labour.

During second stage of labour 12.5-25 mg helps to provide good sedation and effective analgesia.

Higher doses of ketamine (>1 mg/kg) lead to emergent psychomimetic effects and respiratory depression in mother, low APGAR score and rigidity in the neonate.

Regional Analgesia Techniques

- Spinal
- Epidural
- Combined spinal epidural analgesia

They are the most popular methods of pain relief during labour, providing excellent pain relief yet awake and a cooperative patient during labour.

Opioids and local anaesthetics alone can provide analgesia; combining both, results in good analgesia, reduced dose requirements with few maternal and foetal side effects.

Pain of first stage of labour is initially confined to T11-T12 dermatome but later on involves T10-L1 dermatomes as well.

Pain during late first stage and second stage of labour involves the S 2, 3, 4 dermatomes.

Absolute contraindications to regional anaesthesia are:
- Infection over injection site
- Bleeding diathesis; anticoagulant therapy
- Marked hypovolaemia
- Sensitivity to local anaesthetics
- Patient refusal
- Raised intracranial pressure

Relative contraindications are:
- Pre-existing neurological disease
- Disorders of spine
- Cardiac diseases.

Intraspinal Opioids

Preservative free opioids are given intrathecally as a single dose or intermittently via an intrathecal catheter. They are suitable for high risk patients with significant cardiovascular disease such as Aortic stenosis, Fallot's tetralogy, Eisenmenger's syndrome.

Intraspinal opioids do not cause motor blockade and maternal hypotension except Pethidine which has weak local anaesthetic properties.

Intrathecal morphine (0.5-1 mg) produces prolonged analgesia for 6-8 hours during first stage of labour. Onset of analgesia is slow (45-60 minutes) and associated with high incidence of side effects.

Combining morphine (.25 mg) with fentanyl (25 mcg) or sufentanil (5-10 mcg) results in rapid onset (5 minutes) and short duration (4-5 hours).

Intermittent boluses of pethidine 10 mg, fentanyl 5-10 mcg, sufentanil 3-10 mcg via an intrathecal catheter can also provide satisfactory analgesia.

Disadvantages

Incomplete analgesia, lack of perineal relaxation and side effects such as pruritis, nausea, vomiting, sedation and respiratory depression.

Side effects improve with low dose Naloxoane (0.2 mg/hr IV).

Epidural Opioids

Morphine

Higher dose >7.5 mg (high incidence of side effects) of morphine is needed during labour.

Analgesia is more effective for early first stage of labour.

Slow onset (30-60 minutes) but long duration (up to 24 hours) of effect.

Pethidine

Epidural pethidine 100 mg provides good but short duration analgesia (1-4 hours).

Epidural fantanyl (50-200 mcg) or Sufentanil (10-50 mcg) produce rapid onset of analgesia (5-10 minutes) for short duration (1-2 hours) with few side effects.

Combining low dose of morphine (2.5 mg) with Fentanyl (25-50 mcg) or Sufentanil (10-20 mcg) may result in rapid onset and prolongation of analgesia (4-5 hours) with fewer side effects.

Single shot epidurals do not cause neonatal depression; however caution should be exercised following repeated administration.

NARCOTIC DOSAGES FOR RELIEF OF LABOUR PAIN		
Agent	*Epidural*	*Intrathecal*
Morphine	7.5 to 10 mg	0.5 to 1 mg
Pethidine	100 mg	10-20 mg
Fentanyl	50-200 mcg	5 to 25 mcg
Sufentanil	10 to 50 mcg	3 to 10 mcg

Local Anaesthetics

Lumbar epidural anaesthesia and spinal (intrathecal) anaesthesia can be used during labour and delivery. Pain relief for first stage requires block of T10 to L1 sensory level while second stage requires a T10 to S4 block.

Continuous lumbar epidural is most versatile and most commonly used because it can be used for pain relief in the first stage of labour as well as anaesthesia for subsequent vaginal delivery or caesarean section if necessary.

Single shot epidural is used when pain relief is initiated just prior to vaginal delivery.

Epidural Drugs

Local anaesthetics	Dose	Opioid	Comments
Bupivacaine 0.25%	10-15 ml	None	Good analgesia with slight motor blockade
Bupivacaine 0.125%	10-20 ml	Fentanyl 2-4 µgm/ml	Excellent analgesia with no motor block
Bupivacaine 0.125%	10-20 ml	Sufentanil 0.5 µgm/ml	Excellent analgesia with no motor block
Ropivacaine 0.2%	8-15 ml	Fentanyl 2-4 µgm/ml may be added	Excellent analgesia with no mother block

Steps for Epidural Analgesia for Labour Pains

- Preanaesthetic evaluation.
- Explain the procedure to the parturient and record informed written consent.
- Start intravenous fluids through 18 or 20 G IV catheter (preferably non-dextrose containing crystalloids or colloids) and apply appropriate monitors (EKG, pulse oximeter and NIBP).
- H_2 receptor antagonists (Ranitidine 50 mg) + Metoclopramide 10 mg + Ondansteron 8 mg may be administered intravenously.

- Ensure emergency drugs (ephedrine, atropine, etc) and equipment for resuscitation is available.
- Clean and prepare the back of the patient with antiseptic solution. Make a wheal with local anaesthetic at site of puncture (preferably with 26/24 G hypodermic needle at L2/3 or L3/4 level) and inject into interspinous space also.
- Place epidural catheter taking aseptic precautions through Tuohy's needle. Secure catheter well and turn the patient supine.
- Administer test dose of Lidocaine 1.5%, 2 ml or 1.0%, 3ml with epinephrine 1:2,00,000. Watch for signs of intravascular or intrathecal injection.
- Once epidural placement of catheter is confirmed administer initial dose of either Lidocaine 1% or Bupivacaine 0.125 to 0.25% or Ropivacaine 0.125% to 0.175% + Sufentanil 10-15 microgram or Fentanyl 20-25 microgram
- Total volume of 10-15 ml may be required to provide good analgesia.
- Subsequent analgesia options
  a. Intermittent every hourly 8-10 ml or
  b. Continuous infusion 8-12 ml/hour of Bupivacaine 0.125% alone or in combination with Fentanyl 1-2 microgram/ml.
- Check blood pressure frequently every 2 minutes for initial 15 minutes and then every 5-10 minutes till block wears off.
- Treat hypotension aggressively if it occurs. Ephedrine 3-6 mg every 2-3 minutes till systolic blood

pressure is more than 90 mm Hg. Exaggerate uterus displacement towards left, rapid IV fluids, Atropine 0.6 mg may be administered intravenously.

- Maintain patient in lateral position. To avoid lateralization of epidural block turn the patient to the opposite side every 15 -30 minutes.
- Check sensory level prior to every top up and confirm correct placement of epidural catheter prior to top up.

Drug Doses for CSE in Labour

Route	Local anaesthetic	Opioid
Intrathecal injection	Bupivacaine .1 to .25% 1 to 2.5 mg	Fentanyl 20-25 mcg or Sufentanil 3-10 mcg
Epidural top-ups	Bupivacaine .1 to .125%; 10-15 mg first stage labour; usually adequate for second stage and assisted delivery For operative delivery titrate the dose with Bupivacaine .5% or Xylocaine 2%	Fentanyl 20-25 mcg or Sufentanil 5-10 mcg

mcg = micrograms

**Combined Spinal Epidural Analgesia
(Ambulatory Labour Analgesia)**

The aim is to provide analgesia while preserving motor function so as to permit ambulation and improve maternal satisfaction.

1. Locate the epidural place with 16 gauge Tuohy's needle.
2. Pass a 12 cm long, 26-27 gauge spinal needle through it into the subarachnoid space.
3. Inject intrathecally, Bupivacaine 2.5 mg (1 ml of .25%), Fentanyl 25 mcg or Sufentanil 5 mcg, Saline .5 ml; withdraw the spinal needle.
4. Thread an epidural catheter via Tuohy's needle and leave it in epidural space; the needle is withdrawn. The catheter is well secured and used for later supplementation or institution of anaesthesia via epidural route.
5. Observe for 20 minutes the BP, level of sensory and motor block.

   If the block is adequate, the patient is allowed to walk.

   If it is unilateral, turn the patient to unblocked side, give 5 ml of epidural mixture*; then further 10 ml in supine position (Do not repeat dose of subarachnoid injection).

   If inadequate, give epidural injection.

   If there is rectal pressure, give Fentanyl 100 mcg in 10 ml saline via epidural catheter.

The subarachnoid block wears off in 90 minutes; give the first top-up of 15 ml of epidural mixture* via epidural catheter; subsequent top-ups of 10 ml as required.
*Epidural mixture consists of:
Bupivacaine 50 mg (10 ml of .5%) + Fentanyl 100 mcg + Saline to make up the volume to 50 ml.

Patient-controlled epidural analgesia (PCEA) is relatively a new method of maintaining labour analgesia. PCEA has been compared with continuous epidural infusion (CEI). Patients who receive PCEA are less likely to require anaesthetic interventions, require lower doses of local anaesthetic, have less motor block and greater maternal satisfaction than those who receive CEI.

Most appropriate PCEA solutions are Bupivacaine .0625 to .125%, or Ropivacaine 1 mg/ml, 10-15 ml with Fentanyl 3 mcg/ml. On demand boluses are 3 to 5 ml with 10 to 15 minute lockout interval.

Complications of Epidural Analgesia

1. *Maternal hypotension* is one of the commonest complications of epidural analgesia which can compromise uterine perfusion and oxygen transfer to foetus. It can be avoided by pre-loading with 750-1000 ml of Ringer Lactate; in presence of oedema or PET, administration of colloid or less amount of crystalloid may be appropriate. The dose of local anaesthetic is titrated to minimum dose necessary to achieve sensory block only.

If hypotension occurs, it is treated aggressively with Ephedrine 5-30 mg IV.

Bradycardia if observed, is treated with Atropine .6-1.2 mg IV.

If profound hypotension occurs following epidural, determine whether accidental intrathecal injection has occurred.

2. *Accidental dural puncture*: If it occurs, inject a small amount of fentanyl or sufentanil intrathecally; withdraw the needle and reinsert at another place.

3. *Intravascular injection*:"Every epidural injection is intravascular, until proved otherwise." "Every epidural dose should be a test dose".

These two thoughts if kept in mind, will prevent unintentional intravascular injection.Tachycardia immediately following epidural dose is indicative of intravascular injection.

4. *Accidental intrathecal blockade*: Usually intrathecal puncture is recognised by the appearance of CSF. Occasionally it is unrecognised and intrathecal injection of drug occurs resulting in dense motor and sensory block; or the mother experiences unexpected rapid and complete pain relief; in worst case scenario a total spinal may occur.

5. *Inadequate or failed block or atypical block* all can occur. Usually due to the drug being injected at a place other than the epidural or intrathecal space.

6. *Persistant neurological deficit* occurs in 1 in 20,000 cases; temporary deficit is more common. It is wise

not to inject any solution epidurally if pain results. Check the solution, reposition the needle or catheter.

7. *Epidural haematoma* seen in conditions such as prior heparinization, pre-existing coagulopathy, thrombo-cytopaenia from any cause and use of low molecular weight Heparin. Symptoms are segmental pain and paresis continuing after the epidural block is expected to wear off. A neurological consultation and surgery may be needed.

Key Points

1. Among the current methods of obstetric analgesia, regional analgesia (mainly epidural analgesia) is the best because it is most effective and safe.

2. Walking epidural is the most acceptable method to mother and obstetrician, and is associated with least side effects.

3. Systemic analgesia by parenteral opioids, non-opioid painkillers and inhaled anaesthetic agents provide an alternative to regional analgesia but they are less effective and more hazardous.

4. Psychoprophylaxis and physical methods are not potent enough when used alone.

5. Communication and exchange of information between anaesthesiologists, obstetricians and nurses in an ever changing environment of labour and delivery are essential for a perfect outcome.

6. The safe labour analgesia or anaesthesia requires appropriate staff, facilities and proper equipment for patient safety.

Chapter 9

Anaesthesia for Caesarean Section

General anaesthesia (GA) for caesarean section (CS) is no longer the method of choice. Only about 15% of cases are performed under GA and the number is decreasing.

When time is the limiting factor, GA is sometimes necessary because it offers speed of induction, reliability, control and avoidance of sympathectomy-induced hypotension.

The problems associated with GA are related to failed intubation and aspiration of gastric contents. The physiological changes of pregnancy may increase the incidence of failed intubation and its associated maternal morbidity and mortality.

The factors contributing to increased incidence of aspiration of gastric contents include delayed gastric emptying, increased gastric acid secretion, reduced lower oesophageal sphincter tone, reduced intestinal motility, increased intra-abdominal pressure; many of the patients may not be fasting.

Caesarean section may be indicated for variety of obstetric problems. It may be an emergency or an elective procedure. It is important for an anaesthesiologist to modify the anaesthetic plan according to the circumstances.

Preoperative Evaluation

Parturient should be assessed with consideration of emergent situation. Charts should be reviewed.

• Medical history

- Relevant obstetrical history (PIH, gestational diabetes mellitus, uteroplacental insufficiency, placental position, abruptio placentae)
- Previous anaesthetic exposure
- History of drug allergy
- Fasting status
- Relevant investigations (bleeding and coagulation profile, haemoglobin, etc.)
- Airway assessment
- General and systemic examination (Emphasizing haemodynamic status, fluid retention, etc.).

Patient Preparation

Anxiety Relief

Parturients should be informed about the various anaesthesia techniques and their advantages and disadvantages; patient's preferences, if any, should be noted. A little time spent with the patient by an experienced and confident anaesthesiologist alleviates most of anxiety and need for premedication. However, if an anxiolytic is required a small dose of midazolam 0.5-1.0 mg, fentanyl 25 microgram may be administered.

Aspiration Prophylaxis

- *H_2 receptor antagonists* Ranitidine 150 mg given orally night before and on the day of elective caesarean section effectively raises gastric pH and decreases gastric volume. It offers little or no protection against aspiration of gastric contents during induction, if given less than 1 hour preoperative but will be effective at the time of extubation

- *Antacids* A non-particulate preparation such as Sodium citrate 0.3M 15-30 ml given prior to caesarean section raises gastric pH.
- *Antiemetics* Metoclopramide 10 mg IV raises lower oesophageal sphincter tone and promotes gastric emptying; Ondansteron 4 mg slow IV preinduction, reduces the incidence of PONV.

Transportation of Parturient with Foetal Distress

Operation theatre should be in the vicinity of the labour room. The patient should be transported on her side to avoid aortocaval compression. Oxygen should be administered during transport.

Preanaesthetic Preparation

A bolus of 15-20 ml/kg non-dextrose containing crystalloid fluids (Normal Saline/Ringer Lactate) should be infused through 18 or 20 G intravenous catheter. Dextrose containing fluids may stimulate foetal insulin to cause hypoglycaemia in newborn. All appropriate anaesthesia monitoring should be prepared. Emergency drugs to treat hypotension and bradycardia should be prepared. Emergency drugs for general anaesthesia and equipment for difficult airway should be checked.

Regional vs General Anaesthesia Technique

Parameters	Regional anaesthesia	General anaesthesia
Airway control and complications	Not required	May result in major morbidity and mortality
Awake	Awareness may result in anxiety. But it is a pleasure to witness the birth of baby	Mother is not conscious; there is no anxiety
Quickness	Depends upon the infra-structure, individual skill of anaesthetist.	More stable
Haemodynamic stability	With newer strategies (low dose spinal or epidural anaesthesia) reasonable haemodynamic stability can be achieved	

Contd...

Contd...

Parameters	Regional anaesthesia	General anaesthesia
Foetal depression	Not a concern if patient is haemodynamically stable	Although literature reports no detrimental effect on APGAR score, but there is a potential risk
Technical skill	Simple and easy	Tracheal intubation may require good skill in pregnant patients
Drug and equipment related complications	Backache, PDPH, transient neurological symptoms	Awareness, intubation and drug related complications, risk of hyperthermia

Anaesthesia Techniques

1. General anaesthesia
2. Regional techniques
   a. Spinal
   b. Epidural
   c. Combined spinal epidural
   d. Field block.

Often regional technique is chosen these days. Sensory level up to T4 level should be achieved. Epidural anaesthesia through catheter offers advantage of administering predictable level of anaesthesia. In addition, the catheter can be used to provide post-operative pain relief.

Epidural Anaesthesia

Steps for epidural anaesthesia for caesarean section

1. Start non–dextrose intravenous fluids through 18 or 20 G IV catheter.
2. Sodium citrate 0.3M 15-30ml orally and H_2 Receptor antagonists (Ranitidine 50 mg) + Meto-cloperamide 10 mg/+ Ondansteron 8 mg may be administered intravenously if not given earlier.
3. Ensure emergency drugs and equipments for resuscitation and general anaesthesia.
4. Apply monitors (EKG, pulse oximeter, NIBP).
5. Administer oxygen.
6. Place epidural catheter taking aseptic precautions at L2-3 or L3-4 level. Secure catheter well and turn the patient supine with left lateral tilt.
7. Place a wedge under left buttock to displace uterus.
8. Administer test dose of Lidocaine 1.5% 3 ml with epinephrine 1:2,00,000 and watch for signs of intravascular or intrathecal injection.
9. Once correct placement of epidural catheter is confirmed, administer incremental doses of Lidoacine 2% 5 ml or Bupivacaine 0.5% 5 ml every 2-5 minutes till desired level is achieved.

10. Do not exceed 20 ml of local anaesthetic.
11. Administer test dose prior to every top up.

Adjuvants

Adjuvant drugs can be used in addition to local anaesthetics to improve efficacy and duration. Epinephrine added in 1:2,00,000 concentration helps to decrease absorption thus reducing chances of systemic toxicity, intensify the motor block and prolongs the duration of local anaesthetics. Narcotics (fentanyl 25-50 microgram or pethidine 50 to 75 mg) may be added to local anaesthetics to enhance the analgesia. This also helps to provide postoperative analgesia with a lower anaesthetic dosage. Other adjuvants to enhance the epidural anaesthesia include bicarbonates and other local anaesthetics.

Spinal Anaesthesia

Spinal anaesthesia is simple to perform and easy to master. It offers advantage of dense, quick block with minimal failure rate as compared to epidural anaesthesia. Spinal anaesthesia is considered safe and technique of choice for elective as well as emergency caesarean section these days. This has an edge over general anaesthesia in non-fasting and patients with anticipated difficult airway or bronchial asthma.

Steps for spinal anaesthesia for caesarean section:
(Steps 1-5 are the same as for Epidural anaesthesia)

6. Clean and prepare back of patient with antiseptic solution. Make a projection of supine and make a wheal with local anaesthetic, perform lumbar puncture using midline or paramedian approach at L2-3 or L3-4 level with a fine cutting or non-cutting spinal needle (preferably with a Whitacre spinal needle of 26 G or 25 G size). Administer hyperbaric bupivacaine 0.5% 2.0 to 2.4 ml (10-14 mg) or hyperbaric lidocaine 5% 1.0-1.2 ml (50-60 mg). Dose can be adjusted according to height of the patient.

7. Turn the patient supine immediately with left lateral tilt or with a wedge under left buttock to displace uterus away.

8. Table tilt can be manipulated to limit the sensory block to dermatome T4.

9. Treat hypotension aggressively if it occurs. Ephedrine 3-6 mg in increments every 2-3 minutes till systolic blood pressure is more than 90 mmHg. Exaggerate uterine displacement leftwards. Rush fluids. Atropine 0.6 mg may be administered intravenously.

In very severe hypotension delivery of baby may be expedited.

Adjuvants

Epinephrine added in 1:2,00,000 concentration to lidocaine helps to decrease absorption thus prolongs the duration of lidocaine. Opioid addition to local anaesthetics reduces dose required for spinal block.

Bupivacaine 0.5% 1.5 ml + Fentanyl 15 to 20 microgram mixture are sufficient for spinal anaesthesia. This combination not only provides good intraoperative analgesia, prolonged postoperative analgesia but also helps to reduce incidence of hypotension and vomiting.

Combined Spinal-Epidural Anaesthesia for Caesarean Section

Combined spinal-epidural anaesthesia offers merits of both spinal and epidural techniques while covering their demerits. Spinal component provides quick, dense and reliable block whereas epidural catheter helps to supplement an inadequate spinal block, extend anaesthesia if required and provides postoperative analgesia. The presence of epidural catheter permits a low dose of local anaesthetic for spinal anaesthesia, thus minimising chances of consequent hypotension.

Steps for standard combined spinal anaesthesia for caesarean section:
(Initials steps 1-5 are the same as for epidural block/or spinal anaesthesia)

6. Clean and prepare back of patient with antiseptic solution. Place epidural needle. Perform lumbar puncture using needle through needle technique with a long spinal needle of 27 G through epidural needle. Administer hyperbaric bupivacaine 0.5% 1.6 to 2.2 ml (8-12 mg). Fentanyl 15-20 microgram may be added to local anaesthetics. Withdraw the spinal

needle. Then insert epidural catheter through the epidural needle and fix the catheter well.

7. Turn the patient supine immediately with left lateral tilt or with a wedge under left buttock to displace the uterus away.

Steps for sequential combined spinal anaesthesia for caesarean section Sequential Combined Spinal Anaesthesia is indicated in patients requiring precise control of the level of block to perform caesarean delivery. The dose of spinal drug is kept intentionally low and is supplemented with an epidural block.

* All the steps are same as standard CSE except the dosage. Low dose spinal bupivacaine 0.5% 1.2 to 2.0 ml (6-10 mg) is given in sitting position to achieve T8-9 level block only.

* Turn the patient supine immediately with left lateral tilt or with a wedge under left buttock.

* The block is extended to desired level using epidural local anaesthetics in incremental doses (bupivacaine 0.25%).

General Anaesthesia for Caesarean Section

General anaesthesia was a technique of choice for emergency caesarean sections following foetal distress and PIH. But over last two decades, the higher morbidity and mortality due to failed intubation and aspiration of gastric contents, has lead to change in trend. Spinal anaesthesia for caesarean section has become the preferred technique. However GA in caesarean delivery is still used in cases of patient refusal for regional block, severe coagulopathies, acute maternal hypovolaemia, pre-existing cardiac or neurological lesions, infection at or near the site of lumbar puncture, cord prolapse and other causes of foetal distress.

Some of the relative contraindications to use of GA are difficult airway, malignant hyperthermia and bronchial asthma.

Steps for general anaesthesia for caesarean section:

1. Oral administration of 30 ml of Sodium citrate 15-30 minutes prior to induction.
2. H_2 receptor antagonists (Ranitidine 50 mg) + Metoclopramide 10 mg + Ondansteron 8 mg may be administered intravenously if not given earlier.
3. Start intravenous fluids through 18 or 20 G IV catheter (preferably non-dextrose containing crystalloids or colloids).
4. Maintain left lateral tilt or place a wedge under left buttock.
5. Ensure availability of emergency and anaesthesia drugs. Check anaesthesia equipment, oxygen reserve, suction machine and equipment for resuscitation.
6. Apply monitors (EKG, pulse oximeter, $EtCO_2$ and NIBP).

7. Preoxygenate with 100% O_2 for 3 to 5 minutes with a tight fitting mask.

8. Administer thiopentone sodium 4 mg/kg. Apply cricoid pressure and administer immediately succinyl choline 1.0-1.5 mg/kg.

9. Perform laryngoscopy and place 7.0 mm endo-tracheal cuffed tube into trachea once adequate muscle relaxation is achieved. Inflate cuff to just occlude the trachea to prevent leak and aspiration. Start ventilating the lungs; maintain normocapnia.

10. Administer nitrous oxide and oxygen mixture 1:1 or 2:3; 1:3 along with low concentrations of inhalational anaesthetic agent to maintain anaes-thesia. Isoflurane 0.6% or Halothane 0.5% can be used.

11. After delivery of the baby, narcotics should be administered to supplement analgesia. Propofol may be used as an alternative to inhalational anaesthetic agent after delivery of baby.

12. Administer non-depolarising muscle relaxant in low dosages as necessary.

13. Reverse neuromuscular blockade after surgery when there is clinical appreciation of respiratory efforts or there is sufficient recovery on neuro-muscular monitoring if being used.

14. Extubate the patient when fully awake and return of full muscle tone.

Field Block for Caesarean Section

This is the safest anaesthetic technique for CS and at times the only means when general and spinal anaesthetic techniques may not be feasible.

1. Often no premedication is advisable. A tranquillizer such as Midazolam 1-2 mg intravenously may be given beforehand.
2. 80-100 ml of 0.5% lignocaine with adrenaline and hyaluronidase is prepared.
3. With the patient lying first on one side and then on the other the 9th, 10th, 11th and 12th thoracic nerves are each blocked with 2.5 ml of solution as they run beneath their ribs, using a 2.5 cm needle.
4. Next a skin weal is raised over the upper border of the symphysis pubis. A 5 cm needle is then used to infiltrate behind the pubis, along both pubic rami and the insertion of the abdominal rectus muscles using 20 ml of solution.
5. A skin weal is raised in the midline below the umbilicus (for a vertical skin incision). With the 10 cm needle, 20 ml of solution is used to infiltrate subcutaneously and intradermally along the line of the skin incision.
6. The remaining solution is kept until the abdomen has been opened. The peritoneal cavity and uterine surface is sprayed with remaining solution.
7. Opioids may be injected intravenously after delivery of baby to supplement analgesia.

Key Points

Anaesthesia-related complications are a leading cause of pregnancy-related maternal mortality. Difficult or failed intubation following induction of general anaesthesia for caesarean delivery remains the major contributory factor to anaesthesia-related maternal complications. Although the use of general anaesthesia has been declining in obstetric patients, it may still be required in selected cases. Because difficult intubation in obstetric anaesthesia practice is frequently unexpected, careful preanaesthetic evaluation of all parturient should identify the majority of patients with difficult airway and avoid being caught unawares.

Chapter 10

Anaesthesia for Complicated Obstetrics

ANAESTHESIA FOR FOETAL DISTRESS

- Caesarean section for foetal distress is usually considered urgent and an emergency situation; a quick anaesthetic technique is required.
- Spinal anaesthesia and epidural block through previously placed epidural catheter for labour analgesia are often used and safe for emergency caesarean delivery.
- General anaesthesia has been used for years because of its rapidity and fear of maternal hypotension with spinal anaesthesia. However due to increased risk of maternal morbidity related to general anaesthesia, trend has shifted towards the use of spinal anaesthesia for emergency caesarean section. But GA, is still the method of choice for emergencies like cord prolapse and abruptio placenta.

ANAESTHESIA FOR PREGNANCY INDUCED HYPERTENSION (PIH)

- PIH involves 5-10% of all pregnancies and is a treatable cause of maternal morbidity.
- Timing of surgery and type of anaesthesia are important.
- Emergency caesarean delivery for pre-eclampsia is no more an urgent situation as was thought, earlier.
- Meticulous controlling of arterial blood pressure and vital organ perfusion is more important. Expert and aggressive preoperative preparation of the woman

with severe pre-eclampsia ultimately determines her intraoperative outcome.

- General anaesthesia or regional anaesthesia are commonly used methods and can be considered comparable and equally useful.
- There is considerable reduction in maternal morbidity and mortality when using regional anaesthesia, hence it is the preferred technique today.
- However, the management of anaesthesia in patients suffering from preeclamptic toxaemia (PET) has to be selected and tailored individually.
- Time spent preoperatively in fluid volume optimisation, in assessment of ventricular function, filling pressures and systemic vascular resistance, aspiration pneumonitis and seizure prophylaxis, control of hypertension, correction of coagulopathy and on attenuation of presser response is valuable and will have profound effects on the perioperative course. (See also chapter 23 Critical Care in Obstetrics).

MANAGEMENT OF POSTPARTUM HAEMORRHAGE (PPH)

- Postpartum haemorrhage (PPH) happens in 1% of obstetric patients and is usually unexpected.
- Excessive bleeding after delivery may result from uterine atony, disruption of the genital tract, placental abnormalities, coagulation disorders and miscellaneous obstetric complications. Most cases were associated with uterine inertia or placenta accreta.

- Prompt treatment is imperative. Pharmacological treatment includes oxytocics, methyl ergometrine and prostaglandins.
- Patients with previous caesarean section with placenta previa often land up with placenta acreta, leading to postpartum haemorrhage and emergency hysterectomy. It is recommended to proceed with two wide bore IV lines and general anaesthesia in such circumstances.
- Risk of PPH is greater (8.3 times) when there is delay of more than half an hour in administration of prostaglandins after delivery of the baby.
- Use of prostaglandins is associated with significantly more maternal side effects such as gastrointestinal upset, bronchospasm and pyrexia.
- Prostaglandins are less effective when administered orally.
- Prostaglandins can be administered directly intrauterine in cases of caesarean section and as uterine irrigation in vaginal delivery in difficult situations. Although injectable prostaglandins appear to be effective in preventing postpartum hae-morrhage, concerns about safety and cost, limit their suitability for routine prophylactic management of third stage of labour.

Anaesthetic Management in PPH

Rapid transfer to OT can be life saving; any bleeding associated with hypotension and not responding to 500 ml to 1000 ml of fluid resuscitation should be transferred to OT. In cases of significant PPH $\pm$ hypotension $\pm$ surgical indication:

- Send for blood
- Rapid evaluation of anaemia, poor perfusion and early shock
- Review the cause and proposed surgical operation, check BP, HR, JVP
- Obtain large bore IV access, preferably in upper limbs; give IV H_2 blocker and prokinetic agent
- Administer antacids
- Consider placement of CVP line/arterial line for monitoring and inotropes
- If CVS is unstable prepare for general anaesthesia
- If CVS is stable and further bleeding is unlikely, consider using an existing epidural catheter.

General Anaesthesia (Rapid Sequence Induction)

- Opioids (Fentanyl 1-2 microgram/kg)
- Ketamine 1 mg/kg
- Succinylcholine 1.5 mg/kg
- Volatile agents (Isoflurane) or total intravenous anaesthesia (Propofol, Ketamine depending upon haemodynamics).

Regional Anaesthesia (only in Haemodynamically Stable Patient)

- T 7-S 4 saddle block
- Epidural (if catheter *in situ*) lignocaine 2%, 10 ml with epinephrine 1:2,00,000, or Bupivacaine 0.25%

- Spinal (if no coagulopathy) bupivacaine 0.5% 1 ml ± fentanyl 15-25 microgram.

ANAESTHESIA FOR EMERGENCY PERIPARTUM HYSTERECTOMY

- Emergency hysterectomy in obstetric practice is generally performed in life-threatening situations. The rate of peripartum hysterectomy is 1:900 deliveries approximately.
- Many of the caesarean hysterectomies can be avoided if complications leading to these catastrophic situations are treated aggressively in time.
- Resuscitation of parturient is an important and challenging task in these unforeseen circumstances for an attending anaesthesilogist.
- The main indications for hysterectomy are:
  1. Ruptured uterus
  2. Uncontrollable haemorrhage from atonic uterus
  3. Sepsis and morbidly adherent placenta.
- Main goals to be achieved are:
  1. Maintenance of volume status with crystalloids, colloids, blood and blood products.
  2. Monitoring and maintenance of haemostasis.
  3. Monitoring and maintenance of temperature.
  4. Administering anaesthesia.
  5. Providing adequate pain relief.

Chapter 11

Postoperative Care

Recovery from anaesthesia should be ideally a smooth process but is often characterised by airway obstruction, shivering, agitation, delirium, pain, nausea, vomiting and hypothermia/hyperthermia.

Even patients receiving regional anaesthesia can experience marked decreases in blood pressure because the sympatholytic effects of regional blocks prevent compensatory reflex vasoconstriction when patients are moved.

Routine Recovery

Vital signs and oxygenation should be checked on arrival in the postoperative ward. Blood pressure, pulse and respiratory rate are measured every 5 minutes for 15 minutes or until stable; then every 15 minutes.

At least one temperature recording is made.

Monitor oxygen saturation with pulse oximeter continuously in all patients recovering from GA.

All patients recovering from GA should receive 30–40% oxygen; patients with pulmonary dysfunction will need oxygen supplementation for longer period. Patients with COPD and history of CO_2 retention should be nursed in head up position and their oxygen intake needs to be carefully regulated (so as not to wipe out their respiratory drive). Deep breathing and coughing are encouraged.

Patients recovering from regional anaesthesia also need supplemental oxygen because they may be sedated or haemodynamically unstable. Blood pressure should be carefully monitored; bladder catheterization may be necessary after spinal/epidural.

Pain Control

Postoperative analgesia is needed not only for pain relief but there is evidence of a physiological benefit also. Pain causes stress which stimulates the sympathetic nervous system with its adverse effects on the body.

Prolonged pain causes reduced physical activity leading to venous stasis. In a parturient there is already a state of hypercoagulability which coupled with delayed ambulation due to pain, results in increased risk of DVT and pulmonary embolism.

Effective analgesia helps to reduce stress of surgery and haemodynamic fluctuations resulting in smooth postoperative course, early ambulation and discharge.

Pain can be managed with parenteral or intraspinal opioids, epidurals or specific nerve blocks. Analgesia must be adequate but without excessive sedation. When patient is fully awake, patient controlled analgesia can be instituted.

Opioids are most commonly used; titration of small intravenous doses is generally safe (Morphine 2-4 mg or Pethidine 10-20 mg). Analgesic effects usually peak within 4 to 5 minutes but maximal respiratory depression may not be seen till 20 to 30 minutes later. Intramuscular route suffers from delayed or variable onset (10-20 minutes) and delayed respiratory depression (up to 1 hour).

If an epidural catheter is in place, epidural fentanyl (50-100 mcg) or morphine (3-5 mg) can provide excellent pain relief; however delayed respiratory depression with morphine mandates monitoring precautions for 12-24 hours afterwards.

Mild to moderate pain can be managed with analgesics such as Butorphenol 1-2 mg, or Ketorolac tromethamine 15-30 mg or Diclofenac.

Agitation

Before the patient is fully responsive, pain is often manifested as postoperative restlessness; other causes of restlessness are hypoxia, acidosis, hypotension, marked anxiety, fear and adverse drug effects. Treat the cause; if agitation still persists it can be treated with intravenous Midazolam (.5 mg-1 mg).

Nausea and Vomiting

Postoperative nausea and vomiting are common following GA; they can also occur due to hypotension after spinal/epidural anaesthesia. Highest incidence is seen in young women.

Droperidol IV 25 mcg/kg, given intraoperatively reduces the incidence significantly; Metoclopramide (.15 mg/kg) or Ondansetron (.05-.1 mg/kg) are quite effective.

Shivering

It can occur because of intraoperative hypothermia or effects of anaesthetic agents. Hypothermia can result from cold ambient temperature in OT, cold intravenous fluids, cold gases and prolonged exposure. Shivering can follow epidural injection of local anaesthetics; other causes can be sepsis, drug allergy or transfusion reaction.

Shivering in these cases represents body's efforts to increase heat production and raise body temperature; it may be associated with intense vasoconstriction.

Shivering can result in metabolic acidosis, can increase oxygen consumption, CO_2 production and cardiac output significantly. These effects are poorly tolerated by patients with pre-existing cardiac and pulmonary diseases.

Shivering is treated by keeping the patient warm; warming IV fluids before infusion. Small doses of pethidene 10-20 mg IV, or Tramadol can dramatically reduce or stop shivering.

Hypotension

Hypotension results from surgical blood loss, third space sequestration of fluid, ongoing haemorrhage and inadequate volume replacement. Failure of the myocardial pump (commonly due to arrhythmias or pre-existing ischaemic heart disease) may present as hypotension. It can also be an early sign of sepsis or anaphylaxis, both of which cause vasodilatation.

Hypotension is presumed to be due to hypovolaemia until proved otherwise. Volume expansion is usually the first step in the treatment of hypotension in the immediate postoperative period because rapid fluid administration treats most causes and provides the necessary first step before vasopressor therapy.

An indwelling bladder catheter is particularly useful in such circumstances to monitor urinary output.

ECG will reveal irregularities of rhythm or ischaemia.

Elevation of lower limbs augments venous return; colloids and crystalloids can be given at the rate of 10-20 ml/kg while haematocrit is assessed to guide further volume replacement.

Oxygen supplementation is always indicated.

Hypertension and Tachycardia

Several causes of tachycardia and hypertension require intervention but not drug treatment. Bladder distention, hypothermia, shivering, carbon dioxide retention, emergence delirium are common and easily treated causes of postoperative hypertension. In many cases blood pressure elevation >20% of baseline level in the absence of symptoms will resolve without further treatment.

Postoperative pain is a potent stimulus for tachycardia and hypertension which will settle down with adequate analgesia. Tachyarrhythmias, pre-existing hypertensive disease, clonidine withdrawal or compromised cardiac or renal function that may be adversely affected by elevated blood pressure may demand primary treatment by drugs to reduce heart rate and blood pressure.

Treatment options include beta-blockers, ACE inhibitors, calcium channel blockers and direct vasodilators therapy.

Hypoxia

The PaO_2 decreases after GA even when respiratory function appears to be normal; it is influenced by the site of operation, smoking, age, the presence of cardio-respiratory disease and obesity. The hypoxia is caused by ventilation and perfusion mismatch and often corrected by oxygen administration.

Other causes of hypoxia in the early postoperative period are CNS depression because of sedatives or narcotics used as a part of anaesthesia technique, residual neuro-muscular paralysis because of incomplete reversal of the effect of muscle relaxant and respiratory obstruction due to tongue falling back, or presence of secretions, blood or vomitus.

Clearing the airway, administration of oxygen and treating the cause is recommended.

Discharge

- All patients must be evaluated before being sent to the wards.

Postanaesthetic Recovery Score

Colour—O_2 saturation

O_2 saturation > 92% in room air	2
Needs oxygen to maintain O_2 saturation > 90%	1
O_2 saturation < 90% with oxygen supplement	0

Circulation

BP within 20% of normal	2
BP within 20-50% of normal	1
BP deviating >50% from normal	0

Consciousness

Awake, alert, oriented	2
Arousable but drifts back to sleep	1
No response	0

Respiration

Can breathe deeply and cough	2
Shallow but adequate exchange	1
Apnoea or obstruction	0

Activity

Moves all extremities	2
Moves two extremities	1
No movement	0

(Modified from Aldrete JA, Kronlik D: A Post- anesthetic Recovery Score Anesth Analg 1970;49:924)

Ideally the patient should be discharged when the score is 10.

- Observe for at least 30 minutes after the last parenteral dose of narcotic for respiratory depression.
- Other discharge criteria are easy arousability, full orientation, the ability to maintain and protect the airway.
- All vital signs must be stable for at least 1 hour.
- Patients should have the ability to call for help if necessary.
- There should be no surgical complications.
- The patients should be pain free and normothermic.
- Patients receiving regional anaesthesia should show signs of resolution of both sensory and motor blockade.

Key Points

- Analgesia should be provided by multimodal approach; instead of using one drug in high doses, it is safe and efficacious to use multiple drugs to relief pain.
- Pain management can be improved by educating all concerned including nursing staff.
- A subanaesthetic concentration of local anaesthetic administered through epidural infusion is safe and effective way of giving good pain relief.
- Addition of narcotics to local anaesthetics helps to improve quality of analgesia and reduces need of higher local concentrations.
- CSE is preferred technique for anaesthesia during surgery and extending its benefit to provide pain relief in the postoperative analgesia.
- Systemic opioids and NSAIDs can be also used as an alternative.

Chapter 12

Anaesthetic
Emergencies

SUPINE HYPOTENSION

Prevention

1. Identify parturient at risk of developing supine hypotension by:
   - Fall in systolic pressure more than 20 mm Hg in supine position
   - Baseline tachycardia
   - Polyhydroamnios, Twin pregnancy
   - PIH
   - Hypovolaemic patient (Dehydration, Antepartum haemorrhage).
2. Preload with non-dextrose crystalloids 20 ml/kg or colloids 10 ml/kg.
3. Check blood pressure frequently every 2 minutes for initial 15 minutes and then every 5-10 minutes.

Management

1. Treat hypotension aggressively if it occurs. Ephedrine 3-6 mg in increments every 2-3 minutes till systolic blood pressure is more than 90 mm Hg.
2. Exaggerate uterine displacement leftwards.
3. Rapid IV fluids.
4. Atropine 0.6 mg may be administered intravenously diluted in 5 ml normal saline or as such.
5. Maintain patient in lateral position.
6. In intractable hypotension ask the surgeon to deliver the baby (at term).

HIGH SPINAL/TOTAL SPINAL ANAESTHESIA

This may result from inadvertent intrathecal puncture while performing epidural anaesthesia or with barbotage/exaggerated tilt/excessive dose of local anaesthetic in spinal anaesthesia.

Diagnosis

- Hypotension
- Bradycardia
- Loss of consciousness
- Tracheal tug
- Respiratory failure.

Treatment

- Restrict further spread by manipulating table tilt.
- Use vasoconstrictors and inotropes to support blood pressure.
- Atropine 0.6 mg should be administered intravenously and repeat dose may be given if bradycardia persists till maximum dose of 2.4 mg is given.
- Oxygen supplementation.
- Tracheal intubation may be required to support respiration.

INTRAVASCULAR LOCAL ANAESTHETIC INJECTION OR LOCAL ANAESTHETIC TOXICITY

Local anaesthetic toxicity happens in two situations:
1. Accidental intravascular injection while administering epidural or infiltration blocks.

2. Excessive dose administered in a vascular area with high absorption potential.

Clinical Features

- CNS features usually precede CVS depression except bupivacaine which may directly present with ventricular fibrillation.
- Warning signs and symptoms:
  — Numbness of tongue
  — Circumoral tingling, tinnitus
  — Strange visual disturbances and sensations
  — Light headedness and dizziness
  — Tremors
  — Dysarthria.
- Convulsions leading to apnoea and respiratory arrest
- CVS features include hypotension, bradycardia, prolonged PR interval and broad QRS complexes, dysrhythmias, AV block, Ventricular fibrillation or Asystole.

Management

1. Maintain airway.
2. Maintain ventilation and oxygenation.
3. Support haemodynamics: Atropine, mephenteramine, dopamine.
4. Treat convulsions with thiopentone sodium 50-100 mg IV.
5. Bupivacaine induced ventricular fibrillation needs CPR.
6. Reversal of hypoxaemia and acidosis.

FAILED INTUBATION (Figs 12.1 to 12.2)

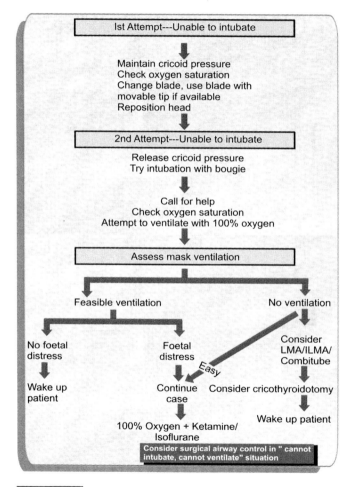

Figure 12.1

Failed intubation drill

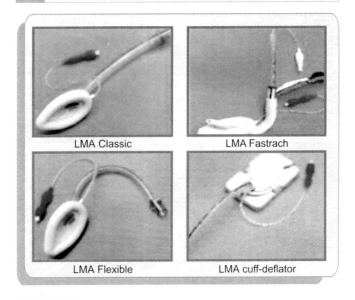

LMA Classic | LMA Fastrach
LMA Flexible | LMA cuff-deflator

Figure 12.2

Various types of LMA

STEPS OF LMA INSERTION (Fig. 12.3)

Step 1 Preparation: Choose the correct size autoclaved sterile LMA. Deflate it completely to make cuff look like a flange and apply lubricant on the back of cuff.

Step 2 Introduction: Induce deep general anaesthesia. Then position head and neck as for tracheal intubation. Hold LMA like a pen with index finger on front of cuff and start introducing it in oral cavity.

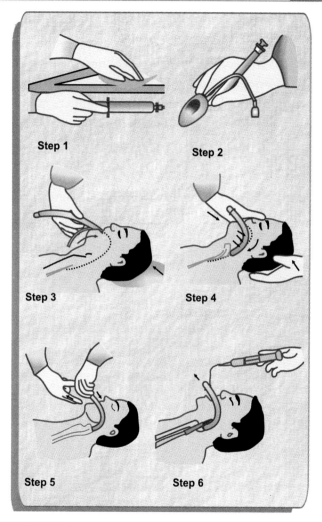

Step 1

Step 2

Step 3

Step 4

Step 5

Step 6

Figure 12.3

LMA insertion

Step 3 Insertion: Try to insert LMA applying pressure on cuff and skid it against hard palate.

Step 4 Insertion: As the mask moves downwards, keep the index finger placed till it is fully introduced to keep epiglottis away from cuff. Keep other fingers out.

Step 5 Placement: Check that the black line on the tube of LMA faces upper lip. Now immediately inflate cuff of LMA.

Step 6 Confirmation: Connect LMA to anaesthetic circuit/ AMBU Bag and check that both lungs expand on pressing the bag.

Avoid inserting with several movements or jerking up and down in pharynx after resistance is felt.

INTRAOPERATIVE PPH

1. Compress uterus bimanually.
2. Administer uterotonics
   - Oxytocin 5-10 units given IV slowly or in infusion is often sufficient to manage third stage of labour. Higher doses and infusion rates may be needed in management of PPH (80 units in 500 ml of Ringer lactate infused over 30 minutes postpartum).
   - Prostaglandin F2α (sulprostone), 500 micrograms, one or two doses administered intramuscularly are sufficient to control PPH in most

of cases with few side effects. Methyl analogue of prostaglandin F2α (Carboprost tromethamine) is freely available in 125-250 microgram snap off ampoules.

3. Uterine and vaginal exploration
4. Initiate timely surgical haemostasis
   - Stepwise uterine devascularisation
     — B-Lynch suture
     — Bilateral hypogastric artery ligation (BHAL) or internal iliac ligation
   - Subtotal or total hysterectomy (Emergency obstetric hysterectomy may be indicated as life saving procedure. It is important to identify the parturient with potential risk for PPH and to prevent morbidity and mortality related to this obstetric problem. Resort to hysterectomy sooner rather than later especially in cases of placenta accrete or uterine rupture).
5. Consider angiographic embolization (ASE).

ANAPHYLAXIS

Anaphylaxis may result from variety of anaesthetic drugs (muscle relaxants, induction agents and local anaesthetics), uterotonics and antibiotics. Prompt and definitive treatment is crucial since mortality increases with delay in management.

Clinical Features

- Urticaria

- Flushing
- Tachycardia
- Hypotension
- Cardiovascular collapse
- Bronchospasm.

Management

1. Discontinue the suspected drug.
2. Discontinue surgery and anaesthesia in grave situations.
3. Call for additional help.
4. Administer 100% oxygen and maintain ABC.
5. Lay the patient supine with legs raised to augment venous return.
6. Administer
   - Adrenaline 50-100 mcg IV over 1 minute for cardiovascular collapse and severe bronchospasm (0.5 to 1ml of 1:10,000 ampoule of adrenaline diluted in 10 ml normal saline)
   - For cardiac arrest, adrenaline can be given in doses of 1 mg IV and pushed with normal saline
   - IV fluids; balanced salt solution 25-50 ml/kg
   - Hydrocortisone 100-500 mg bolus;
     1-2 gm Methylprednisolone
   - Antihistaminics:
     Chlorpheniramine 10-20 mg slow IV
     Diphenhydramine 0.5-1 mg/kg
     Consider H_2 antagonists

7. Perform arterial blood gas analysis
   Consider Bicarbonate 0.5-1 mmol/kg if there is persistent hypotension or acidosis.

8. Infusion of adrenaline or nor-adrenaline may be needed to support haemodynamics for some time. Adrenaline 4-8 mcg/min (5 mg adrenaline in 500 ml saline gives 10 mcg/ml).
   Nor-adrenaline 4-8 mcg/min (4 mg Nor-adrenaline in 500 ml dextrose gives 8 mcg/ml).

9. Bronchodilators may be needed for persistent bronchospasm.

10. Do not attempt any investigation until immediate treatment has been completed. Approximately 1 hour after beginning of reaction, take 10 ml of blood in a plain glass tube and store at 20°C; send to lab. to estimate serum tryptase concentration.

    - If the patient has received spinal/epidural block, higher doses of adrenaline may be needed.
    - Use of adrenaline may alter uteroplacental perfusion which may adversely effect the foetus.
    - Difficult intubation is more likely in pregnant patient. The associated angioedema because of anaphylaxis may further compromise the airway. Endotracheal intubation should be performed at the first sign of respiratory distress.

OLIGURIA (Fig. 12.4)

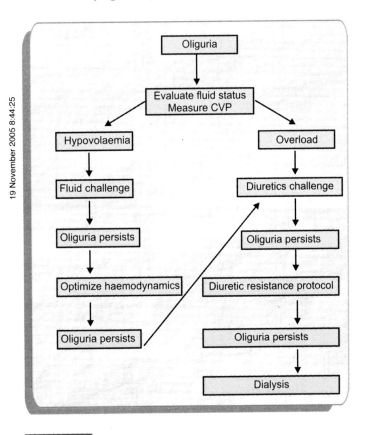

Figure 12.4

Flow chart to manage oliguria

INTRAOPERATIVE DESATURATION (Fig. 12.5)

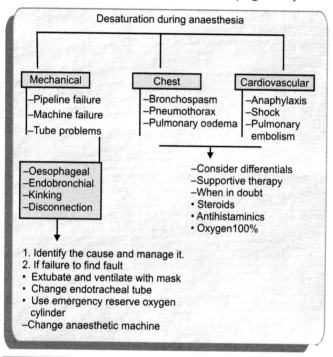

Causes and management of desaturation

HYPERGLYCAEMIC KETOACIDOSIS

Lack of insulin and excess of glucagons in IDDM type I results in accumulation of free fatty acids (acyl CoA) in hepatic cells with incomplete enzymatic conversion to carbon dioxide and water, thus there is excess of acetyl CoA and other ketoacids.

Management

Fluids and Electrolytes

1. In severe diabetic ketoacidosis approximate losses are: Water 5-10 L, sodium 400-500 mmols and potassium 250-700 mmols.
2. The fluid loss is hypotonic as urine sodium is always less than 55 mmol/L.
3. Mostly patient in DKA are hyper- or normokalaemic, but they have always net potassium deficit which gets unmasked during fluid resuscitation.
4. Fluid and electrolyte therapy should be adjusted to individual needs rather than a strict protocol.
5. Establishment of circulating volume with normal saline or colloids at times is the first line of treatment, thereafter it be substituted with hypotonic half strength saline.
6. It is important to be cautious about overhydration as it may lead to cerebral or pulmonary oedema especially in patients with renal and cardiac compromise.
7. Potassium should be supplemented only after the primary resuscitation with fluids has been achieved.

Insulin Therapy

1. Hyperglycaemia should be corrected gradually. Insulin infusion is better in correcting acidosis.
2. Insulin infusion should be continued even after achieving normoglycaemia and should be supple-

mented with glucose containing solutions possibly at higher glucose levels as there may be insufficient glucose and insulin to shift glucose intracellular.

Other Issues

1. Bicarbonate therapy should not be used unless there is severe acidosis, i.e. pH < 7.20 or BE- ECF less than 12 mmols/L (deficit > 12 mmols/L).
2. Nasogastric tube should always be placed as gastric emptying is delayed in DKA and labouring parturient.
3. Antibiotics are given only if there is strong clinical suspicion of infection. There can be mild leucocytosis without evidence of infection in DKA.
4. Abdominal pain of DKA should not be dismissed as a part of DKA syndrome.
5. Magnesium and calcium supplementation should be made appropriately.

HYPEROSMOLAR HYPERGLYCAEMIC NON-KETOTIC COMA

More common in NIDDM or type II diabetes mellitus. Coma more frequent and with higher mortality.

1. Thrombotic events are more frequent and heparin therapy may be instituted if there is no contra-indication.
2. Hypotonic saline resuscitation should be slow (2-3 days).

3. Low dose insulin therapy should be instituted.
4. Too aggressive a therapy, predisposes to more complications of treatment.

HYPERTENSIVE EMERGENCIES

Seen in parturient with PIH, preexisting essential hypertension, inadequate depth of anaesthesia and pheochromocytoma.

Management

1. Treat the underlying cause.
2. Antihypertensive drugs:
   - Hydralazine 5-10 mg slow IV; and may be repeated after 20 minutes
   - Nifedepine 5-10 mg sublingually or intranasal (Not recommended these days)
   - Labetalol 25-50 mg slow IV, repeated every 5 minutes to maximum of 200 mg.
3. Short acting drugs may be administered through infusion
   - Esmolol: Loading dose 500 microgram over 2 minutes, then infusion 50-200 microgram/min
   - Lindolol: a newer drug seems to be promising
   - Nitroglycerine 25-0.5 microgram/kg/min
   - Sodium nitroprusside 0.25-0.5 microgram/kg/min.

ECLAMPSIA

Prevention

Aggressive management of preeclampsia and hypertension is the key to prevent seizures.

Management

1. Magnesium Sulfate: Loading dose is 6 gm of $MgSO_4$ over 20-30 minutes followed by infusion 2-3 gm/hour for 24 hours. Another bolus of 2-4 gm may be repeated in case convulsions reoccur. Watch for side effects such as hypotension and oliguria.
2. Whenever treating a patient with $MgSO_4$, patient must be observed for loss of tendon reflexes ($MgSO_4$ levels of 10 mEq/L), myocardial depression ($MgSO_4$ levels of 10-15 mEq/L), respiratory failure ($MgSO_4$ levels of 12-15 mEq/L) and cardiac arrest at 25-30 mEq/L.
3. Episode of convulsions may be terminated by a small dose of thiopentone sodium (50-100 mg) administered intravenously.
4. Diazepam (5-10 mg) IV slow over 2-5 minutes may be sufficient to terminate episode of seizures while waiting for $MgSO_4$ to have its effect.
5. Cerebral and visual disturbances often resolve spontaneously in few days after control of preeclampsia and delivery.

PULMONARY OEDEMA

1. Identify the mechanism.
   - Hydrostatic

- Capillary leakage
- Idiopathic or unexplained.

2. Find the cause:
   - *Hydrostatic*: Fluid overload, LV failure, cardio-myopathy, tachyarrhythmias, preexisting valvular lesions (mitral stenosis)
   - *Capillary leakage*: Aspiration syndrome, amniotic fluid embolism, anaphylaxis, trauma, severe sepsis, pancreatitis
   - *Idiopathic or unexplained*: Neurogenic.

Management

1. Treat the underlying cause.
2. Monitoring: Vitals, EKG, oxygen saturation, pulmonary capillary wedge pressure (PCWP) (in frank non-resolving pulmonary oedema).
3. Oxygenation.
4. Restrict fluids.
5. Diuretics: Loop diuretics.
6. Morphine sulphate 3-5 mg slow IV or S/C.
7. Ventilation and PEEP may be required in patients who are not maintaining oxygen saturation.

CARDIOPULMONARY RESUSCITATION (CPR)

Main concerns, which demand attention during cardiopulmonary resuscitation of pregnant woman, are difficulty in performing CPR and risk of hypoxia to two lives—mother and foetus.

Initial resuscitation efforts require increased fluid push and left lateral tilt to prevent supine hypotension syndrome.

Newer Modifications in CPR Protocols

1. Early BLS (Basic Life Support) and early defibrillation has been emphasised for the best outcome of survival as the most of patients are in VF or pulseless VT.
2. Early Defibrillation is a priority (if available) as it is the only effective method of terminating VF (Ventricular Fibrillation). Precordial chest compressions are next.
3. Intravenous access and tracheal intubation are also recommended early in ACLS (Advanced Cardiac Life Support).
4. Choice of vasopressors: Repeated adrenaline administration has not shown better neurological outcome after resuscitation. Vasopressin 40 units single dose is recommended as an alternative.
5. Checking of carotid pulse to establish a diagnosis of cardiac arrest is deferred as it is difficult even for an experienced person to appreciate a carotid pulse; look for signs of circulation, instead.

THE CHAIN OF SURVIVAL

Early access to emergency services

↓

Early BLS

↓

Early defibrillation to reverse VF

↓

Early advanced life support to stabilise

Sequence of Actions

- Ensure safety of rescuer and victim
- Check for responsiveness—shake and shout
  - If responds—let victim be in safe position; assess the need of help
  - If does not respond—Call for help
- Open airway
  - Head tilt (Avoid head tilt if suspected neck injury)
  - chin lift
- Check breathing (Look, Listen and feel for 10 sec)
  - If she is breathing more than occasional gasp—keep on side/recovery position and watch
  - If she is not breathing, then give rescue breaths with 2 consecutive breaths
  - If there is difficulty in giving breaths, check inside of the mouth and clear the obstruction, if any
- Look for movement/signs of circulation
- Check the carotid pulse for not more than 10 sec (it is not necessary in the latest guidelines)
  - If there are signs of circulation—continue giving rescue breaths if necessary
  - If there are no signs of circulation—start chest compressions 100/minute
- Combine rescue breathing and compressions 15 compressions: 2 consecutive breaths.

Continue resuscitation till return of signs of life or qualified help reaches or you become exhausted.

Anaesthesia Related Morbidity and Mortality

Problem	Incidence	Cause	Treatment	Comments
Backache	Majority (75%) of women during and after pregnancy report backache. Incidence is about 50% from 24th week onwards. It declined to 37% after a year of delivery. Of the females whose backache persisted for a year, 29.8% had an epidural block and 26.3% had no block	There is no direct association between epidural analgesia and postpartum backache except the first day after delivery. Relaxin hormone has been strongly implicated	NSAIDs

Weak narcotics

Extensor group exercises | Previous history of backache is the only factor associated with persistent back pain (PBP). |
| Postdural puncture | It is a common complication of | CSF leak | NSAIDs
Weak narcotics | The availability of fine and pencil tip |

Contd....

Contd....

Problem	***Incidence***	***Cause***	***Treatment***	***Comments***
headache (PDPH)	spinal anaesthesia. Incidence has been minimised to less than 10% with the use of fine spinal needles. Unintentional dural puncture (UDP) during labour after epidural analgesia is an infrequent occurrence in hands of an experienced anaesthetist		Plenty of fluids. Bed rest. However, whenever UDP occurs, which often results in PDPH, epidural blood patch (EBP) may be given in the same sitting. Another EBP may be required in some patients after about a week. Recently intravenous cortisone has been tried successfully to treat PDPH.	needles has overcome the need for postoperative foot up position as was required earlier. It is established fact that splitting rather than cutting the longitudinal director dural fibres with spinal needle results in lower incidence of PDPH
Transient neurological symptoms (TNS)	Reported incidence of TNS is as high as 37%	5% hyperbaric lignocaine The other drugs implicated are	Self limiting and spontaneous relief after 24-72 hours	Avoid hyperbaric lignocaine 5% for caesarean delivery

Contd....

Contd....

Problem	Incidence	Cause	Treatment	Comments
		procaine, prilocaine and mepivacaine. In a recent study in parturients, hyperbaric bupivacaine, which was earlier thought to be free of TNS, has been implicated to cause TNS (8.8%) after spinal anaes-thesia		
Nausea and vomiting	It is a commonly seen unpleasant experience in the	Patient charac-teristic, type of anaesthesia,	Unfortunately nothing has worked well, probably due to	The latest practice of using low dose local anaesthetics

Contd....

Contd....

Problem	Incidence	Cause	Treatment	Comments
	parturient under-going caesarean delivery in the intra-and post-partum period	narcotics, haemodynamics, fasting status, pregnancy and labour, have been known to cause PONV	multifactor genesis of PONV. Prokinetic drug, Metoclopramide 10 mg may be administered prior to transfer to OT. Newer antiemetic, 5 HT3 receptor antagonists have been tried alone and in combination with variable success rate. Dexamethasone 8 mg combined with 4 mg of ondansteron had been found to be more effective than the individual drug. Oxygen administered intraoperatively has	and opioids for spinal anaesthesia result in stable haemodynamics

Contd....

Contd....

Problem	Incidence	Cause	Treatment	Comments
			been found to reduce the incidence of intra and postpartum nausea and vomiting	
Failed tracheal intubation and aspiration pneumonitis	Barnardo PD and Jenkins JG reported incidence of failed tracheal intubation as 1/249 in 8970 obstetric general anaesthetics. Second major complication is aspiration pneumonitis.	There is substan-tial evidence that there is improve-ment in acid peptic disease (APD) during pregnancy. However, the margin of pH safety is lost in peripartum period. James CF, et al found pH less than 2.5	A dose of ranitidine night before and one hour prior to surgery can be given as prophylaxis against acid aspiration. During labour, to ensure safety, patient may be given HT3 antagonist and 30 ml of 0.3 M of sodium citrate prior to emergency caesarean section. Nevertheless,	Labouring patients may be allowed to have clear fluids. For elective caesarean delivery and non-obstetrical surgery, patients should be advised fasting orders as for other routine surgeries

Contd....

Contd....

Problem	Incidence	Cause	Treatment	Comments
		in most of his cases in the peripartum period	precautions such as rapid sequence induction and prophylaxis against aspiration are recommended	
Awareness during general anaesthesia	Rare occurrence in anaesthesia for non-obstetrical surgery, but more commonly seen in caesarean delivery under GA	Awareness during general anaesthesia for caesarean section was of great concern in the past as anaesthesiologist's tendency to avoid narcotics and anaesthetics with fear of respiratory depression in the newborn	A median BIS 60 or below should be maintained	Recently, Yeo SN studied depth of anaesthesia using BIS monitoring should be used in parturient for caesarean delivery being conducted under general anaesthesia

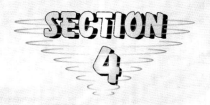

SECTION 4

ANAESTHESIA AND MEDICAL DISORDERS OF PREGNANCY

Chapter 13

Pregnancy and Cardiovascular Disease

Cardiac disease complicates 1-2% of pregnancies. Although rheumatic heart disease remains the most common cause of heart disorders presenting during pregnancy, recent advances in medical and surgical care allow more women with congenital heart disease to reach child bearing age and become pregnant. Some females may get cardiac disease as a complication of pregnancy. The anaesthesiologist must be aware of the cardiac disease and its effect on pathophysiology during various stages of pregnancy and labour. Good maternal and foetal outcome depends upon rational management of obstetrics and obstetrical anaesthesia.

CARDIOVASCULAR CHANGES DURING PREGNANCY

General:
   Blood volume increases approximately 50%
   Systemic vascular resistance falls approximately 20%
   Blood is hypercoagulable
   Cardiac output increases 30 to 45%
   Stroke volume increases early in pregnancy
   Heart rate increases by 10 to 15 bpm, peaking in 3rd trimester

Intrapartum:
   Cardiac output increases by additional 15% with each contraction
   Blood pressure increases by 10 to 20 mm Hg
   Cardiac output increases 60% immediately after vaginal delivery
   Haemodynamic changes are less pronounced and cardiac output is higher in lateral supine position
   Haemodynamic variables are less labile with conduction anaesthesia blocking the pain-stress cascade

Contd....

ECG changes:

QRS axis shifts 15 degrees to left
Low voltage complexes may be present
Ectopic beats more common
Bouts of supraventricular tachycardia more frequent

Principles of Management

- Cardiac disease during pregnancy is best managed by team approach of obstetrician, anaesthesiologist and cardiologist, beginning at an early stage of pregnancy.
- Risk stratification is done on the basis of NYH association functional classification.
- Structural cardiac lesion needs appropriate antibiotic prophylaxis.
- Caesarean delivery is reserved for obstetrical indications only.
- Optimal labour analgesia, helping the mother with forceps or vacuum extraction of foetus and cutting short the second stage, brings rewards.
- Anaesthesia management includes understanding of cardiac lesion and its pathophysiology during pregnancy, appropriate anaesthetic strategy and its skillful execution.
- Invasive monitoring is done only when indicated. Pulmonary artery catheter should be reserved for very sick patient only.

- Adequate postoperative pain relief results in reduced cardiac stress and early ambulation.

Antibiotic Prophylaxis for Subacute Bacterial Endocarditis

Oral	Amoxicillin	3 gm 1 hour before operation and 1.5 gm 6 hours after initial dose
Parenteral	Ampicillin + Gentamicin	2 gm IM or IV 30 minutes before operation 1.5 mg/kg (not to exceed 80 mg) IM or IV 30 minutes prior to operation
	Ampicillin/ Amoxicillin + Gentamicin	1.5 gm 6 hours after initial dose of Ampicillin
Alternative parenteral regimen for patients allergic to penicillin, amoxicillin	Vancomycin + Gentamicin	1 gm infused over 1 hour beginning 1 hour before surgery 1.5 mg/kg (not to exceed 80 mg) IM or IV 30 minutes prior to operation

Strategy for Valvular Cardiac Pathology

Lesion	Heart rate	Preload	Contractility	After load	Rhythm	Comments
Mitral stenosis	Low (80-100)	N/↑	N/↑	N	Important	1. Avoid AF with fast ventricular rate 2. Avoid sudden hypotension/reduction in SVR 3. Avoid factors leading to pulmonary hypertension 4. Avoid chronotropic drugs
Mitral regurgitation and mitral valve prolapse	Higher (100-120)	↑	N/↑	↓	—	1. Avoid increase in SVR 2. Avoid myocardial depression

Contd...

Contd....

Lesion	Heart rate	Preload	Contractility	After load	Rhythm	Comments
Aortic stenosis	N	↑	N	↑	Important	1. Avoid sudden hypotension/reduction in SVR
						2. Avoid hypovolaemia
Subvalvular aortic stenosis	N	↑	↓	N	—	1. Avoid sympathomimetic drugs
						2. Avoid hypovolaemia
Aortic regurgitation	Higher	↑↑	↑	↓	—	
Complex valvular disease	1. Give importance to dominant cardiac lesion and try to understand pathophysiology and compensatory mechanisms.					
	2. Optimal heart rate, preload and after load.					
	3. Try to maintain around baseline values of parameters.					
	4. Avoid sudden increases and decreases in SVR.					

CONGENITAL HEART DISEASE

Congenital heart disease is classified as producing either left to right shunt (Acyanotic heart disease) or right to left shunt (cyanotic heart disease) or an obstructive lesion. It is important understand the pathophysiology of lesion and palliative/corrective surgery performed. Repair of simple shunt lesion results in an almost cured anomaly. Complex shunt lesion may result in new problems. Many patients after these cardiac procedures may have a low threshold for dysrhythmias.

Strategy for Congenital Cardiac Anomaly

L→R SHUNT (VSD, ASD, ETC)

1. L→R shunt leads to pulmonary overflow and these patients are prone to pulmonary congestion when over hydrated.
2. Patients with pulmonary hypertension are prone to reversal of shunt.
3. Avoid hypoxia, hypercarbia and very high inflation pressure during ventilation.
4. Avoid air filled syringe to identify epidural space while performing regional block.

R→L SHUNT
(TETRALOGY OF FALLOT, EISENMENGER SYNDROME)

1. R→L shunt leads to systemic hypoxaemia.
2. Increases in right sided pressures result in increase in shunt fraction.
3. Avoid hypoxia, hypercarbia and very high inflation pressure during ventilation.
4. In patients with variable dynamic pulmonary obstruction, sympathomimetic activity increases the obstruction resulting in worsening of situation.
5. Avoid air filled syringe to identify epidural space while performing regional block.

OBSTRUCTIVE LESIONS
(PULMONIC STENOSIS, COARCTATION OF AORTA)

1. Increases in right sided pressures result in increased CVP and low cardiac output state.
2. Avoid hypoxia, hypercarbia and very high inflation pressure during ventilation.
3. In patients with variable dynamic pulmonary obstruction, sympathomimetic activity increases the obstruction resulting in worsening of situation.
4. Maintain normal or near normal heart rate, preload and after load.

Key Points

1. Compulsively maintain uterine displacement; reductions in preload and increases in after load may be catastrophic.
2. Use saline to identify the epidural space.
3. Avoid epinephrine containing local anaesthetics for test dose as intravenous injection may result in undesirable tachycardia.
4. Labour analgesia using intravenous patient controlled analgesia with fentanyl is a reasonable choice if there is a contraindication to regional analgesia.
5. Supplement oxygen, it is always beneficial and at least not harmful.
6. Maternal and foetal survival is best when perimortem section is performed within 10 minutes.

Chapter 14

Pregnancy, Asthma and Anaesthesia

Classification of Severity of
Chronic Stable Asthma

Type	Symptoms	Night time symptoms	Lung function
Mild intermittent	Symptoms $\leq$ 2 times a week. Asymptomatic and normal PEF in between exacerbations	< 2 times a month	FEV$_1$ or PEF $\geq$ 80% predicted
	Exacerbations brief (few hours to few days); intensity may vary		PEF variability $\leq$ 20%
Mild persistent	Symptoms > 2 times a week, but < 1 time a day	> 2 times a month	FEV$_1$ or PEF > 80% predicted
	Exacerbations may affect activity		PEF variability 20-30%

Contd...

Contd...

Type	Symptoms	Night time symptoms	Lung function
Moderate persistent	Daily symptoms; Daily use of inhaled short-acting beta 2-agonist drugs Exacerbations affect activity. Exacerbations $\geq$ 2 times a week, may last days	> 1 time a week	FEV_1 or PEF > 60% to < 80% predicted PEF variability > 30%
Severe persistent	Continuous symptoms. Limited physical activity. Frequent exacerbations	Frequent	FEV_1 or PEF 60% predicted. PEF variability > 30%

FEV_1 = Forced expiratory volume in 1 second
PEF = Peak expiratory flow
Adapted from National Asthma Education and Prevention Program. Expert Panel Report 2: Guidelines for the Diagnosis and Management of Asthma—National Institutes of Health Pub No. 97-4051. Bethesda, MD, 1997

Things to be Remembered in Acute Asthma

1. Mortality from life threatening acute asthma is high and is often avoidable by early, aggressive therapy.
2. Severe acute asthma patients may be divided in two groups:
   - Insidious deterioration leading to exhaustion.
   - Acute catastrophic bronchospasm with early asphyxiation.
3. Patients with marked 'morning dipping' are at risk of sudden acute catastrophic attacks.
4. The following features on admission are ominous signs and suggest an early requirement for mechanical ventilation:
   - Pulsus paradoxus > 30 mm Hg.
   - Heart rate > 110/min.
   - Silent chest, feeble respiratory effort, cyanosis
   - Deteriorating consciousness level, exhaustion and coma.
   - PEFR < 35% of predicted normal.
   - ABG analysis-rising $PaCO_2$ level, metabolic acidosis.
   - Previous history of severe asthma requiring mechanical ventilation.
5. Medical therapy
   1. A high $PaCO_2$ in acute asthma is not a contra-indication to high FiO_2 therapy.
   2. Treatment of both bronchospasm and inflammation is required.

3. Patients who develop respiratory muscle fatigue can avoid mechanical ventilation with cautious use of CPAP to reduce the work of breathing.

4. Cautious CPAP in patients with a raised FRC may not raise FRC further.

5. Careful attention to hydration is required to avoid mucus plugging.

6. If inhaled agonists, anticholinergics and theophyllines fail to secure improvement, the use of ketamine or halothane as a bronchodilator may be helpful in mechanically ventilated cases.

6. Mechanical ventilation

1. Patients are likely to require additional humidification for removal of inspissated secretions.

2. Excessive air-trapping should be avoided since it is associated with increased risk of pneumothorax, poor left and right ventricular function by distortion of the RV and septum.

3. Pulmonary distension is reduced by accepting moderate hypercapnia:

- Low frequency ventilation (6-10/min)
- Low tidal volume (6-10 ml/kg)
- Low inspiratory flow rates
- Prolonged expiratory time
- Avoid high peak airway pressures (> 50 cmH$_2$O)
- Adequate sedation
- Muscle relaxants to overcome respiratory drive.

MANAGEMENT OF ACUTE ASTHMA
DURING PREGNANCY

1. Oxygen-highest flow rate and concentration should be used.

2. Nebulized Beta 2 agonist bronchodilators: 5 mg salbutamol or 10 mg terbutaline up to 3 doses in first 60-90 minutes; then every 1-2 hours until adequate response.

3. High dose steroids—used in patients who are already on steroids or those who respond poorly during the first hour of treatment. Intravenous methyl prednisolone 1 mg/kg every 6-8 hours. Reduce dose as patient improves.

4. Measure blood gases and rule out pneumothorax by ultrasonography or X-ray chest (If there is strong indication only).

5. Consider intravenous Aminophylline (only if patient requires hospitalization). To be used 6 mg/kg as a loading dose, 0.5 mg/kg/hr initial maintenance dose and then adjust rate to keep blood-theophylline level between 8-12 microgram/ml.

6. Consider SC Terbutaline 0.25 mg if patient not responding to above therapy

(Adapted from recommendations of NAEP Report of the Working Group on Asthma During Pregnancy)

Anaesthetic Considerations during Pregnancy

Key Points

- Determine the efficacy of treatment and ensure optimal pulmonary status preoperatively.
- Pain and hyperventilation of labour can precipitate bronchospasm.
- Narcotics can relieve pain, but can result in respiratory depression and bronchospasm due to histamine release.
- Beta-blockers, ergometrine, prostaglandins especially $PGF_{2\alpha}$ can lead to bronchospasm.
- Regional blocks are safe for obstetrical interventions in controlled asthmatic parturient.
- Acute bronchospasm may contraindicate regional technique due to paralysis of abdominal muscles.
- General anaesthesia requires adequate depth of anaesthesia, avoidance of histamine releasing drugs, smooth and skillful induction and emergence to prevent bronchospasm.
- If bronchospasm occurs, treat aggressively with beta agonists, aminophylline, inhalational anaesthetic agents and maintenance of oxygenation with high concentrations of oxygen.

SEVERE ACUTE ASTHMA

Goals of Therapy

a. To correct hypoxia
b. To alleviate bronchospasm and optimize airflow
c. To avoid maternal exhaustion and progression to respiratory failure.

Management Protocol

a. Administer supplemental oxygen.

b. Begin bronchodilator therapy with inhaled albuterol.

c. Assess FEV_1/PEFR; if greater than 75% of predicted or personal best and no symptoms or wheezing, can discharge to follow-up in clinic.

d. If there is no rapid or sustained relief after 30 to 60 minutes, or if there are signs or symptoms of life-threatening asthma, draw arterial blood gases and begin parenteral corticosteroids (2.0 mg/kg hydrocortisone IV bolus or equivalent, followed by 2.0 mg/kg every 4 hr).

e. If airflow or oxygenation is still severely compromised, add ipratropium bromide 0.5 mg via nebulizer.

f. If still progressing to respiratory failure and intubation appears imminent, give 2 gm IV bolus of magnesium sulfate over 2 minutes, followed immediately by inhaled albuterol and ipratropium.

g. Endotracheal intubation should be performed when, despite maximal pharmacologic therapy, the following exists or occurs:

   1. Inability to maintain a PaO_2 of greater than 60 mm Hg with 90% hemoglobin saturation despite supplemental oxygen.
   2. Inability to maintain a PCO_2 less than 40 mm Hg.
   3. Evidence of maternal exhaustion.
   4. Worsening acidosis despite intensive bronchodilator therapy (pH< 7.2-7.25).
   5. Altered maternal consciousness.

Critical Laboratory Tests

a. Arterial blood gases
b. FEV_1, PEFR
c. Chest X -ray, Sputum Gram stain.

Consultation

Respiratory therapy, pulmonary medicine, and intensive care medicine.

Chapter 15

Pregnancy, Anaemia and Anaesthesia

High proportion of women in both industrialised (18%) and developing (35 to 75%) countries become anaemic during pregnancy.

Definition

WHO defines anaemia in pregnancy as a haemoglobin concentration of less than 11 gm dl^{-1} or haematocrit < 0.33 in first and third trimester. In the second trimester a fall of 0.5 gm dl^{-1} due to raised plasma volume is allowed and a cut off value of 10.5 gm dl^{-1} or haematocrit < 0.32 is used.

KINETIC CLASSIFICATION OF ANAEMIA

Excessive Destruction or Loss of Erythrocytes

- Blood loss
  — Acute
  — Chronic.
- Extracorpuscular haemolytic disease
- Antibodies
- Infection (malaria, etc.)
- Splenic sequestration and destruction
- Associated disease states, e.g. lymphoma
- Drugs, chemicals and physical agents
- Trauma to red blood cells—prosthetic valves
- Intracorpuscular haemolytic disease
- Hereditary
  a. Disorders of glycolysis

   b. Faulty synthesis or maintenance of reduced glutathione
   c. Qualitative or quantitative abnormalities in synthesis of globin
   d. Abnormalities of red cell membrane
   e. Erythropoietic porphyria.
- Acquired
   a. Paroxysmal nocturnal haemoglobinuria
   b. Lead poisoning.

Inadequate Production of Mature Erythrocytes

Deficiency of Essential Substances

- Iron
- Folic acid
- Vitamin B_{12}, C
- Other vitamins
- Protein.

Deficiency of Erythroblasts

- Atrophy of bone marrow: aplastic anaemia
- Infiltration of bone marrow
- Endocrine abnormality
- Chronic renal disease
- Chronic inflammatory diseases
- Infections
- Collagen diseases
- Cirrhosis of liver.

Anaesthetic Considerations

Oxygen Flux

Denotes the oxygen delivery per minute to tissues and is equal to:
Cardiac output × Haemoglobin concentration 1.39 ×% Saturation of haemoglobin/100.

Preoperative Check up

History

Mild anaemic patients may be asymptomatic or may present with a history of lassitude, dyspnoea, dizziness, easy fatigue or irritability.

Severely (Hb < 8 gm/ dl) anaemic parturient may complain of palpitation due to increased cardiac output, which may precipitate angina and heart failure especially during labour. History of drug intake, such as salicylates, is important.

Clinical Examination

Complaints of breathlessness, oedema over feet, pallor, and signs of increased cardiac output (tachycardia, wide pulse pressure, systolic ejection murmur or signs of cardiac failure).

Mental disturbances and subacute combined degeneration of the cord may be the feature of Vit B_{12} deficiency.

These findings should be carefully noted in the history sheet to avoid false allegation on administration of anaesthesia in the postoperative period.

Features of chronic renal failure (contribution to anaemia due to insufficient production of erythropoietin) or endocrine dysfunction (inadequate production of thyroid hormone) should be looked for.

Basic Data for Evaluation

Haematological
- Haematocrit
- Haemoglobin
- Red cell indices
- Total and differential leucocyte count
- Platelet count
- Reticulocyte count
- ESR
- Peripheral blood film.

Other Investigations
- Urine analysis
- Stool for occult blood, ova, cysts
- Serum creatinine
- Serum bilirubin
- Serum ferritin.

Administration of Anaesthesia

a. *Regional anaesthesia*: Spinal or Epidural technique will need preloading which may further decrease Hb and may precipitate heart failure. Thus in anaemic parturient, after infusing 500 ml of crystalloid fluid it is logical to switch on to vasoconstrictor to sustain the blood pressure and to replace blood loss intravenously with colloids or blood depending upon the severity of anaemia and blood loss. Patients with megaloblastic anaemia (Vitamin B_{12} deficiency) may develop neurological symptoms postoperatively. So, regional anaesthesia should preferably be avoided in these cases as it may be blamed for the neurological complication.

b. *General anaesthesia*

Following precautions prevent many undesirable problems:

- Adequate preoxygenation to prevent hypoxia during intubation
- Slow administration of intravenous induction agents
- A CVP line is preferable if a fair amount of blood transfusion is contemplated
- Avoid undue hypothermia and hyperventilation (alkalosis) to prevent shift of oxygen dissociation curve. Alkalosis impairs oxygen delivery and hypocapnia reduces cardiac output
- Cyanosis is a late sign and its absence does not necessarily indicate adequate oxygenation in anaemic patients
- Spontaneous ventilation with high concentration of inhalational agents may depress respiration and myocardial performance, both of which are essential for maintenance of adequate oxygen flux.

- Mild tachycardia and wide pulse pressure may be physiological and should not be confused with light anaesthesia.
- Care should be taken to control the airway
- Timely and adequate replacement of blood.
- Tissue perfusion should be monitored clinically and by ABG analysis if required

Special Situations

Sickle Cell Disorders

1. Patient should be well hydrated.
2. Patient with a 'steady state' of chronic haemolysis has a haemoglobin level of 6-9 gm/dl. This level of haemoglobin is well tolerated by the patient with HbS which has a lowered oxygen affinity than HbA. Any attempt to raise the level of haemoglobin will increase the blood viscosity leading to possibility of crisis.
3. Red cell enriched with 2,3 DPG displaces oxygen dissociation curve to the right as a compensatory mechanism.
4. Hypoxia is to be avoided at all costs in order to prevent crisis. Some authorities recommend 50% oxygen during anaesthesia.

Thalassaemias

1. Apart from Hb estimation, platelet count and prothrombin time should be checked.

2. Iron overload (due to increased absorption from GI tract) and repeated transfusion may lead to functional abnormalities in the liver, endocrine system and the heart (supraventricular dysrhythmias, congestive cardiac failure, pericarditis, etc.).

Postoperative Care

- Extubation should be done when the effect of relaxant has worn off as these patients cannot tolerate hypoxaemia.
- In addition to routine monitoring, vitals should be monitored to catch early the complications of severe anaemia such as heart failure.
- High concentrations of oxygen enriched air should be given by venti mask/mask with reservoir.
- Shivering should be avoided and treated with adequate warming of IV fluids, keeping the patient warm, injection pethidine, etc. as shivering causes a many fold increase in the oxygen requirement.

Chapter 16

Pregnancy and Diabetes Mellitus

Diabetes is the most common medical problem during pregnancy.With the introduction of insulin and strict control of IDDM pregnant patients, maternal and neonatal prognoses have improved considerably. Maternal morbidity is related to hypoglycaemia, keto-acidosis, hypertension, exacerbation of nephropathy, and retinopathy.

The incidence of diabetes in the offspring of IDDM parturients varies between 1 and 3%. The risk is greater (6.1%) if father has IDDM; it is highest (20%) if both parents have IDDM.

It is estimated that of all diabetic pregnancies, 90% are due to gestational diabetes mellitus.

Detection of Diabetes Mellitus

The new diagnostic cut off value of plasma glucose level is 126 mg/dl.

Commercially available dip-stick may be used to identify glucosuria. However this may yield false positive results due to lactose and augmented glomerular filtration rate. Nonetheless the detection of glucosuria warrants further investigation.

PREGNANCY AND DIABETES

Maternal glycaemic control is important in IDDM parturients and glycosylated haemoglobin is a good indicator for this purpose. It has important implication for foetal oxygenation (increased levels are associated with decreased foetal oxygen saturation and decreased P_{50} values). Hence, in parturients with uncontrolled diabetes, foetal oxygenation will be impaired.

Classification of Diabetes Mellitus during Pregnancy

Class	Onset	Fasting glucose levels (mg/dl)	2-hour postprandial glucose levels (mg/dl)	Therapy
A1	Gestational*	< 105	< 120	Diet
A2	Gestational*	> 105	> 120	Insulin

Class	Age of onset	Duration	Vascular disease	Therapy
B	Over 20	< 10 years	None	Insulin
C	10-19	10-19 years	None	Insulin
D	Before 10	> 20 years	Benign retinopathy	Insulin
F	Any	Any	Nephropathy	Insulin
R	Any	Any	Proliferative retinopathy	Insulin
H	Any	Any	Coronary artery disease	Insulin

*When diagnosed during pregnancy: 500 mg or more proteinuria per 24 hour urine collection measured before 20 weeks gestation. Adapted from American College of Obstetrics and Gynecology (1986)

Diabetic ketoacidosis (DKA) is a major cause of foetal morbidity and mortality. Diabetic parturients are at risk of developing diabetic ketoacidosis early, due to changes in insulin requirement, omission of insulin doses, tocolytic therapy with beta-mimetic drugs, use of glucocorticoids to promote foetal lung maturation, excess secretion of stress hormones and high metabolic rate. Preeclampsia is more common in diabetic parturients, the incidence increasing with the severity of diabetes. Preeclampsia is more difficult to diagnose, especially in presence of diabetic nephropathy with associated hypertension.

Diabetic nephropthy is associated with hypertension in 30% of cases in first trimester and as many as 75% by time of delivery. Perinatal outcome will be poor if serum creatinine is >1.5 mg /dl, urinary protein excretion is >3 gm /24 hours and high mean arterial pressure >107 mm Hg.

Diabetic autonomic neuropathy can get worse and cause postural hypotension; gastrostasis is common in diabetic parturients.

ANAESTHETIC CONSIDERATIONS

* Altered uteroplacental blood flow: There is reduction of 35-45% *in utero* placental blood flow in diabetic parturient. A further decrease in placental perfusion due to raised blood sugar, anaesthetic agents and techniques can significantly affect the foetus.
* Hypotension should be avoided as uteroplacental flow is compromised in diabetic mothers.

- Buffering capacity to handle acid load is decreased in newborns of diabetic mothers.
- Diabetic parturient are prone to severe hyperglycaemia and ketoacidosis.
- Prolonged fasting in labouring parturient should be avoided because of accelerated starvation.
- It is safe to administer combined solutions of glucose and insulin.
- Stiff joint syndrome poses difficulties in tracheal intubation due to involvement of small joints of head and neck.
- Regional block is safe for painless and caesarean delivery as it also blunts adrenergic response of adrenals.
- Preloading with non-dextrose fluids should be done prior to regional block.

Anaesthetic Management

Decreased uteroplacental perfusion is the most important change that takes place in diabetic parturient. The foetus of uncontrolled IDDM mother will be hypoxic because:
- Increased maternal glycosylated haemoglobin
- Hyperglycaemia and hyperinsulinaemia
- Significantly decreased uteroplacental perfusion.

Hence hypotension due to regional anaesthesia or vena caval compression must be prevented.

For Labour and Delivery

- Moderate pain relief can be obtained by IM or IV narcotics in early part of labour.
- Lumbar epidural or CSE anaesthesia will provide excellent pain relief both for labour and delivery.
- Continuous epidural infusion of low concentration of local anaesthetic mixed with fentanyl can be used without adverse foetal effect.

  Advantages of epidural pain relief:
  - Decreased maternal catecholamine concentration (following pain relief) leading to increase placental perfusion
  - No maternal hyperventilation and no respiratory alkalosis due to pain relief, resulting in better placental blood flow
  - Less acidosis in foetus.

For forceps delivery 2% plain lignocaine provides dense perineal analgesia.

Close attention to maternal blood pressure is important; if mother is already receiving insulin mixed with 5% dextrose, a second IV line will be beneficial for volume expansion with non-dextrose solution.

Continuous foetal heart rate monitoring is essential throughout labour.

In the absence of an epidural, spinal anaesthesia can be used for forceps delivery. Maternal hypotension must be treated aggressively with volume replacement and use of vasopressors.

PREGNANCY AND DIABETES MELLITUS

Caesarean Sections

The problems in IDDM parturient include utero-placental insufficiency, associated foetal hypoxia, diabetic neuropathy, cardiomyopathy and diabetic scleroderma.

Because of these changes, parturients will be more prone to hypotension, which will be difficult to treat particularly in the severely diabetic.

The infant of mothers who received regional anaesthesia are more acidotic than those whose mothers received GA. The acidosis is related to maternal diabetes and hypotension. If maternal blood glucose is well controlled, volume expansion with Ringer's Lactate is done and maternal hypotension is aggressively managed, then the fetal outcome is similar, under both GA and spinal.

Spinal Vs Epidural

Spinal anaesthesia is the preferred method for caesarean section unless contraindicated. But because of rapidity of onset, the incidence of hypotension is higher following spinal anaesthesia. It may be compounded by the presence of cardiomyopathy and autonomic neuropathy in a severely diabetic parturient. In such circumstances, epidural may be a better choice (Inject the drug slowly).

CSE technique can also be safely used.

GA in diabetic parturients is associated with delayed gastric emptying, limited atlanto-occipital joint extension in patients with diabetic stiff joint syndrome and impaired hormone responses to hypoglycaemia during sleep.

IDDM parturients may be in a better condition to undergo caesarean section under regional than under general anaesthesia. The advantages are that the patients can vocalize signs of hypoglycaemia; also the cardiovascular responses to hypoglycaemia may be blunted under GA.

PERIOPERATIVE MANAGEMENT OF DIABETES MELLITUS

Management depends upon the type of DM, status of current diabetic control and type of surgery.

Aims and Objective

1. To avoid hypoglycaemia.
2. To avoid ketoacidosis.
3. To avoid hyperglycaemia, osmotic diuresis and dehyration.
4. To avoid infection.
5. To improve tissue healing.

Key to good perioperative management of diabetes mellitus is frequent monitoring of blood glucose level and proper dosing of insulin.

Diet Controlled

- Check fasting or Random blood sugar.
  Well controlled: Treat as normal
  Poorly controlled:
  Postpone case and start regular Insulin and Glucose.
  In case of emergency surgery, start with Dextrose
  5% or Dextrose 10% 125 ml/hour and insulin on
  sliding scale.

Sliding Scale Insulin Infusion

Blood sugar level (mmol/L)	Insulin infusion (units/hour)
< 4	0
4.1-9	1
9.1-11	2
11.1-17	3
17.1-28	4
>28	6

Sliding scale infusion is easy, simple and economical
for postoperative use.

1. Add 50 units Insulin to 50 ml of normal saline
   (Insulin 1 unit/ml) for syringe infusion pumps; add
   50 units insulin to 250 ml of normal saline for
   infusion via a drip set.
2. As insulin is administered separately, risk of
   hypoglycaemia stands.

3. Intravenous fluid: Administer 100 to 125 ml of 10% Dextrose. In case of prolonged use or if required to restrict volume to allow administration of other fluids, higher concentration of glucose may be used.

4. Add 20 mmol of potassium per litre of dextrose in this regimen. Increase potassium to 30 mmol/L if potassium levels < 4.0 mmol/L; stop potassium additions if potassium levels are more than 5.0 mmol/L.

ORAL HYPOGLYCAEMIC AGENTS

• Check fasting or Random blood sugar.

Well controlled: Stop sulphonylureas and pyroglutazone one half life prior to surgery (Often need to be omitted on the day of surgery).

• Stop metformins at least 24 hours prior to surgery.
• Start orally after surgery in case of minor procedures.
• Postoperatively, start with glucose and insulin on sliding scale in case of major surgery.

Poorly controlled

• Postpone case and start regular Insulin and Glucose.
• In case of emergency, start with Dextrose 5% or Dextrose 10% 125 ml/hour and insulin on sliding scale.

Insulin Dependent Diabetes Mellitus

• Check 24 hours blood sugar profile.

Well controlled: Omit morning dose of regular insulin/ half dose of intermediate acting insulin and omit long acting insulin on evening prior to surgery.

Start with Dextrose 5% or Dextrose 10% 125 ml/hour and insulin on sliding scale.

- Start orally after surgery in case of minor operation.
- Continue with glucose and insulin on sliding scale in case of major surgery.

Poorly controlled

- Postpone case and start regular Insulin and Glucose.

In case of emergency, start with Dextrose 5% or Dextrose 10% 125 ml/hour and insulin on sliding scale.

Gestational Diabetes Mellitus

- Check 24 hours blood sugar profile and get blood sugar level prior to caesarean section.
- Adjust insulin doses as per table given on page 192.
- Start with Dextrose 5% 125 ml/hour and insulin on sliding scale.
- Continue with glucose and insulin on sliding scale in postoperative period.

Intraoperative Blood Glucose Control

Vellore regimen can also be used for simple, effective and safe control of intraoperative blood glucose.

For every 1 to 50 mg/dl increase in blood glucose concentration more than 100 mg/dl, 1 U of insulin is added to 100 ml measured volume set containing 5% dextrose in water. Hourly monitoring of blood glucose is performed.

Intrapartum Maternal Glycaemic Management

Plasma capillary glucose level (mg/dl)	Insulin infusion rate (IU of regular insulin)	Fluid therapy
< 80	No insulin	Dextrose 5% 125 ml + Ringer lactate
80-100	0.5	Dextrose 5% 125 ml + Ringer lactate
100-140	1.0	Dextrose 5% 125 ml + Ringer lactate
141-180	1.5	Normal saline/Ringer lactate
181-220	2.0	Normal saline/Ringer lactate
> 220	2.5	Normal saline/Ringer lactate

Diabetic Ketoacidosis

It is a major cause of foetal mortality and morbidity. The causes are:

1. Changes in insulin requirement in presence of infection.
2. Omission of insulin doses.
3. Tocolytic therapy with beta mimetic drugs.

4. Use of glucocorticoids to promote maturation of foetal lung.

DKA occurs due to lack of insulin or excess of glucagon. Hyperglycaemia initiates osmotic diuresis leading to dehydration. K^+ and Na^+ concentration are decreased due to osmotic diuresis. Increased concentration of beta oxidative enzymes in liver metabolize free fatty acids to ketone bodies which decrease maternal pH and stimulate respiratory centre. Intracellular K^+ is replaced by H^+ ions and thus total body potassium is depleted. Loss of maternal plasma volume decreases cardiac output and blood pressure ultimately leading to cardiovascular collapse and shock.

Diabetic parturients can develop DKA with blood glucose levels as low as 200 mg/dl.

Clinical Features

1. Anorexia, nausea, vomiting, tachycardia.
2. Polyurea, polydipsia.
3. Abdominal pains or muscle cramps.

In severe cases there is Kussmaul hyperventilation; hypotension and oligurea due to severe hypovolaemia; lethargy due to coma; normal or cold body temperature; fruity odour in breath.

Management

Fluids and Electrolytes

1. In severe diabetic ketoacidosis, approximate losses are: Water 5-10 L, sodium 400-500 mmols and potassium 250-700 mmols.

2. Volume replacement is done with two IV lines, one for rapid fluid infusion and the other for insulin administration.

3. Initial replacement is with normal saline (15-20 ml/kg/hr); approximately 1 lit/hour for 2 hours; accurate monitoring of urine output is essential. From third hour onwards, the fluid rate is reduced to half the previous rate depending on urine output and clinical situation.

4. When the blood sugar is reduced to 250 mg/dl, normal saline is replaced with 5% dextrose in DW.

5. Intravenous fluids should be continued till the patient is able to drink adequate amount of fluids by mouth and there is no nausea.

Insulin Therapy

1. Insulin should be started early and given intravenously; 10 units bolus and then 5 to 10 units per hour.

2. DKA patients exhibit insulin resistance. If hyperglycaemia and anion gap do not show improvement within 2 hours, insulin infusion rates are doubled to overcome resistance.

Other Issues

1. Bicarbonate therapy should not be used unless there is severe acidosis and pH < 7.10 or BE- ECF less than 12 mmols/L (i.e. more deficit than 12 mmols/L).

2. Most patients in DKA are apparently hyper- or normo-kalaemic, but they always have net potassium deficit which get unmasked during fluid resuscitation. Potassium should be supplemented only after the primary resuscitation with fluids has been achieved.

3. Antibiotics are needed only if there is strong clinical suspicion of infection. There can be mild leucocytosis without evident infection in DKA.

4. Magnesium and calcium supplementation should be made appropriately.

5. Nasogastric tube should always be placed as gastric emptying is delayed in DKA and labouring parturient

Hyperosmolar Hyperglycaemic Non-Ketotic Coma

More common in NIDDM or type II Diabetes Mellitus. Coma is more frequent with higher mortality.

1. Thrombotic events are more frequent and heparin therapy may be instituted if there is no contra-indication.

2. Hypotonic saline resuscitation should be slow (over 2-3 days).

3. Low dose insulin therapy should be instituted.

4. Too aggressive therapy predisposes to more complications.

Chapter 17

Coagulation Problems and Anaesthesia

Pregnancy is a hypercoagulation state and there is always a threat of thromboembolism to the mother. Deep vein thrombosis (DVT) and pulmonary embolism (PE) are separate but related aspects of the same dynamic disease process known as venous thromboembolism. There is predominance of venous thromboembolism in the postpartum period.

Indications for Anticoagulant Therapy during Pregnancy

1. Patient with established DVT diagnosis
2. Patients with prosthetic valves
3. Cardiac dysrhythmias-atrial fibrillation
4. Patients at high risk of developing thrombotic and clotting disorder.

Treatment during Pregnancy

- Unfractionated heparin (UFH) is the commonest therapy, as it does not cross uteroplacental blood barrier, has least teratogenicity or haemorrhagic complications. However, mothers do get side effect like thrombocytopenia and osteoporosis.
- In the case of recent thrombosis, delivery should be planned during the time in which anticoagulation therapy has been stopped or minimized.
- Patients with acute DVT of lower limb at risk of developing pulmonary embolism can be advised temporary vena cava filter during pregnancy.

Prophylaxis during Pregnancy

- Prophylactic doses of UFH can be used to reduce the risk of recurrent thromboembolic events in pregnancy.
- Although there are reports indicating safe use of low molecular weight heparin (LMWH) during pregnancy, American College of Chest Physicians (ACCP) consensus constraint the use of LMWH during pregnancy.
- Antithrombotic prophylaxis is recommended from 12 to 36 weeks of pregnancy in high-risk group.
- Low-dose aspirin can reduce the risk of recurrent pre-eclampsia by about 15%, but the role of UFH and LMWH in the prevention of recurrent miscarriage or obstetric complications associated with uteroplacental insufficiency is still uncertain.
- Another subset of pregnant patients who require antithrombotic prophylaxis is antiphospholipid syndrome.
- Use of oral anticoagulants is often restricted in pregnancy due to risk of developing embryopathy.

Anticoagulants and Anaesthesia

- Therapeutic doses of LMWH contraindicate the use of regional anaesthesia.
- A switch to intravenous UFH before delivery allows greater flexibility.

- Epidural and spinal anaesthesia may be used provided the coagulation profile is monitored. Currently the strict protocol has been relaxed. However, procedure should be performed under controlled conditions. It is recommended that type of anaesthesia should be chosen, weighing the potential risks and benefits of various techniques.
- Postoperatively patient should be screened as soon as the effect of regional block wears off to assess for

ANTICOAGULANTS AND NEURAXIAL BLOCKADE

1. Stop oral anticoagulants 4-5 days before neuraxial blockade; prothrombin time (PT) and international normalized ratio (INR) must be measured before initiation of block.
2. PT/INR should be monitored daily and checked before catheter removal, if the anticoagulant dose was given more than 36 hours before the block.
3. Catheter should be removed only when INR is < 1.5.
4. In spite of normal PT / INR, concurrent use of drugs like aspirin, NSAIDs, UFH and LMWH, ticlopidine, clopidogrel may increase the risk of bleeding complications in patients on oral anticoagulants.
5. For patients on prophylactic doses of LMWH wait for 12 hours after the last dose before a neuraxial block. In case of therapeutic doses wait for 24 hours.
6. Postoperatively, first dose of LMWH is given 24 hours after surgery; remove the epidural catheter atleast 2 hours before the dose of LMWH.
7. If epidural catheter is needed for postoperative analgesia, then it is removed 10 to 12 hours after the last dose of LMWH; subsequent dose of LMWH is given 2 hours after the catheter removal.
8. UFH should be given atleast 4 hours before neuraxial block or atleast 30 minutes after removal of catheter.

any new development of neurological deficit. Laminectomy should be carried at the earliest (with in 6-12 hours) if there is any haematoma causing neurological deficit.

• Adequate neurological monitoring is essential during postoperative recovery. Overall, the final decision to use regional anaesthesia in patients receiving drugs that alter haemostasis must be made on an individual basis after assessment of both, the benefits obtained and risks taken (Figs 17.1 to 17.4).

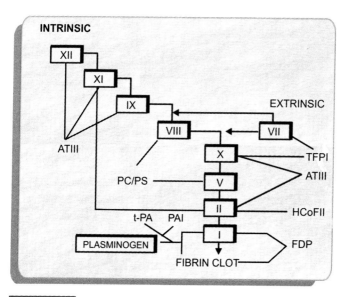

Figure 17.1

New concept of coagulation physiology

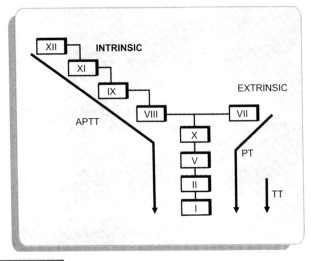

Figure 17.2

Schematic diagram of common laboratory tests

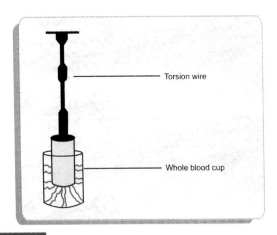

Figure 17.3

Showing diagrammatic principle of thromboelastography

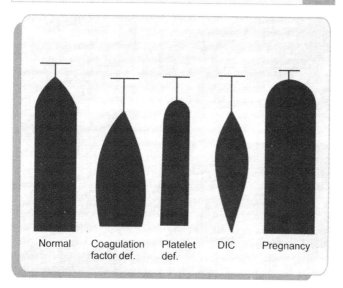

Normal   Coagulation   Platelet   DIC   Pregnancy
         factor def.   def.

Figure 17.4

Showing diagrammatic shapes of thromboelastography graphs of some coagulation states

Things to be Remembered

Neuraxial blockade should ideally be avoided in patients with altered coagulation profile. However, in view of the high risk of complications related to general anaesthesia, the following guidelines are provided for safe placement of epidural catheters:

Unfractionated Heparin

Anaesthesia should be started at least 4 hours after administration of this drug or 30 minutes before, provided pulmonary arterial pressure is normal.

Low Molecular Weight Heparin

This should be administered 12 hours before or 12 hours after the placement of epidural catheter.

Oral Anticoagulants

Provision of regional anaesthesia depends mainly on International Normalized Ratio monitoring.

It is equally important that removal of catheters should follow criteria similar to those listed above for placement of epidural catheter.

HELLP SYNDROME

HELLP syndrome is an acronym for haemolysis, elevated liver enzymes and low platelet count. About 10% of parturients having severe pre-eclampsia and eclampsia are affected by it.

Symptoms include epigastric and right upper quadrant pain (because of subcapsular or intrahepatic haemorrhage), nausea and vomiting. Signs of hypovolaemia and shock suggest intraperitoneal rupture.

HELLP syndrome can be diagnosed by criteria defined by Sibia:

Serum bilirubin levels > 1.2 mg/dl

Elevated liver enzymes

- Lactate dehydrogenase (LDH) levels > 600 U/L
- Aspartate Aminotransferase >70 U/L

Platelet count < 100 000/mm3.

Although peripheral blood smear is a non-specific investigation, it still remains a sensitive diagnostic aid.

Thromboelastogram (TEG), a whole blood visco-elastic coagulation screening test, can be helpful to assess these patients as it measures all phases of co-agulation and fibrinolysis differentially in a single sample of blood.

Maternal mortality is significant. Serious compli-cations include DIC, abruptio placenta, acute renal failure and pulmonary oedema.

Severe persistent shoulder or epigastric pain in case of HELLP syndrome indicates sub-capsular hepatic hae-matoma. There is always risk of rupture and possible vascular collapse.

Management

- In an asymptomatic patient with stable haemo-dynamics and coagulation profiles, no active management is required except control of arterial pressure and monitoring of foetal growth and maternal well being. Normal vaginal delivery may be conducted once gestational age is beyond 32-34 weeks. Before 30 weeks' gestational age caesarean may be indicated, as often this period is associated with prolonged labour.

- Definite management includes delivery; severe disease calls for prompt delivery.

- Early plasma exchange may be considered as an adjuvant therapy in severe and progressive post-partum HELLP syndrome.

- Intraperitoneal capsular rupture can be diagnosed by abdominal paracentesis, ultrasound and abdominal CT. Immediate treatment of hypovolaemia by volume expansion, correction of coagulopathy and management of other aspects of pre-eclampsia is essential.

Key Points

1. Platelet count above 20000/mm^3 is sufficient in asymptomatic patient for vaginal delivery, but platelet count more than 100000/mm^3 is desirable for caesarean section.
2. Platelet packs should be transfused as well as kept ready for caesarean section if count is less than 50000/mm^3.
3. The type of anaesthesia depends upon the coagulation status and the anaesthesiologist's personal judgment. Spinal anaesthesia can be used safely if coagulation profile is normal.
4. The coagulopathy that accompanies HELLP syndrome should not be assessed only before taking the decision on anaesthetic technique, as the condition can be progressive and can become more severe after the epidural puncture is performed.
5. The patient's condition should be observed closely until coagulation normalises.
6. Removal of the epidural catheter must wait until coagulopathy is resolved.
7. Patients with coagulation abnormalities need to be assessed individually. Spinal puncture for anaesthesia is certainly a better choice as compared to placing the epidural catheter for regional block.
8. Blood component therapy should be considered in symptomatic and patients with very low count of platelets.

Chapter 18

Anaesthesia for Obese Parturient

Obesity is defined as excess of body fat, frequently resulting in impairment of health. Obesity in women is present when body mass index (BMI) is greater than 27.3.

(BMI = Weight (kg) divided by height in meters^2)
Normal BMI = 25
Overweight = BMI between 26 to 29
Morbid obesity = BMI > 35 or twice the ideal body weight.

Obesity is associated with the following:

- Diabetes
- Hypertension
- COPD
- Pickwickian syndrome
- Pre-eclampsia
- Liver disease
- Thromboembolism.

Obesity is associated with 'large for date' babies and caesarean delivery. Both general and regional techniques are technically difficult and are associated with complications. The obese patients have a smaller proportion of body water and muscle mass and greater proportion of fat to body weight.

Important body changes in obese parturient are:

- Increased blood volume and cardiac output

- Increased alpha-1 acid glycoprotein leading to increased drug binding sites
- Deranged liver and renal function may alter drug biotransformation.

Maternal Mortality Associated with Pregnancy

Group 1: Mortality < 1%
- Atrial septal defect
- Patent ductus arteriosus
- Pulmonic/tricuspid disease
- Tetralogy of Fallot, corrected
- Bioprosthetic valve
- Mitral stenosis, NYHA class I and II.

Group 2-Mortality 5-15%
2A
- Mitral stenosis, NYHA class III and IV
- Aortic stenosis
- Coarctation of aorta, without valvular involvement
- Uncorrected tetralogy of Fallot
- Previous myocardial infarction
- Marfan's syndrome with normal aorta.

2B
- Mitral stenosis with atrial fibrillation
- Artificial valve.

Group 3-Mortality 25-50%
- Pulmonary hypertension
- Coarctation of aorta, with valvular involvement
- Marfan's syndrome with aortic involvement.

RISKS INVOLVED IN OBESITY

MATERNAL

Obstetric causes
Aspiration
Haemorrhage
Thromboembolism/stroke

Caesarean delivery
Increased blood loss
Prolonged operative time
Difficult epidural placement
Respiratory complications (atelectasis, pneumonia)
Wound infection/dehiscence

Foetal risks
Increased perinatal mortality
IUGR
Low Apgar scores
Low birth weights
Neonatal/childhood obesity
Macrosomia
Increased admission to neonatal ICU

Obesity and Cardiopulmonary Function

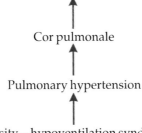

Diminished lung volumes/capacities
Decreased lung/chest wall compliance

↓

Decreased breathing efficiency/gas exchange
Relative hypoxia

↓

Pulmonary shunt

↓

Cardiac compensation

↓

Increased blood/plasma volume
(obesity and pregnancy)

↓

Cardiac work/L efficiency

↓

Ischaemia/infarction

CARDIORESPIRATORY FAILURE

↑

Cor pulmonale

↑

Pulmonary hypertension

↑

Obesity—hypoventilation syndrome
(Pickwickian syndrome)

OBESITY AND PREGNANCY: INTRAPARTUM AND POSTPARTUM MANAGEMENT

Obesity-related problem	Potential solution
1. Difficult peripheral IV access	Central IV line
2. Inaccurate or difficult blood pressure monitoring	Arterial line
3. Pre-existing cardio-pulmonary disease	Continuous electrocardiography, ABG, chest radiography, pulse oximetry
4. Increased risk of general anaesthesia; difficult regional anaes-thesia in emergency	Prophylactic epidural catheter placement
5. Difficult intubation	Regional anaesthesia Prophylactic epidural Awake intubation (Fibreoptic), Failed Intubation Drill
6. Aspiration risks	– Prophylactic epidural – H_2 antagonists (ranitidine 50 mg IV 6-8 hrly and 45 min before surgery) – Sodium citrate (30 ml of 0.3 M) before anaesthesia

Contd...

Obesity-related problem	Potential solution
	– Metoclopramide (10 mg IV over 1-2 min and 45 min before surgery – NPO status in labour
7. Thromboembolic risks	Low-dose heparin (5000 U SC q8-12 hr) Elastic antithrombotic hose (thigh-high) Sequential pneumatic compression boots Early postoperative ambulation Minimize operative/ immobilization times
8. Endometritis/wound infection	Prophylactic antibiotics before incision Thorough skin preparation Pelvic/wound irrigation with antibiotics Surgical drains If Pfannenstiel's incision-maintain—dry surgical site post-operatively

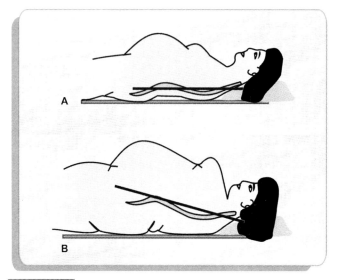

Figure 18.1

Diagram showing spine alignment in (A) Normal parturient, (B) Obese parturient (Note short neck and protuberant breast in obese parturient also)

Key Points

1. Morbidly obese patients have a high incidence of antenatal medical disease, increasing likelihood of maternal and foetal complications.

2. Intrapartum complications and a high incidence of failure of labour to progress increase the likelihood of caesarean delivery. Nearly 50% of labouring morbidly obese patients undergo caesarean section.

3. Because of risk of overdose in these parturient, it is advisable to calculate the drug dosage as per lean body mass rather than absolute body weight. As it is cumbersome to calculate

lean body mass, following equation may be used to calculate ideal body weight:

$$IBW = 25 \times 1.77^2$$

4. General anaesthesia is a major contributor to maternal mortality and should be used as a last resort to save mother or foetus.

5. Early involvement of anaesthesia team and adequate preoperative assessment of these patients is vital. Preoperative assessment includes review of medical record, a careful physical examination, assessment of airway, cardio-respiratory reserve and baseline laboratory screening.

6. *Monitoring*: Pulse oximetry is mandatory during regional and general anaesthesia. Appropriate sized blood pressure cuff is required to monitor NIBP. In very obese parturient, intra-arterial blood pressure monitoring, is recommended.

7. There are reports indicating successful management of caesarean deliveries in morbidly obese parturient using extra long epidural needle. Spinal anaesthesia with long needle has also been used successfully. CSE may be more promising in view of its safety and flexibility.

8. Early epidural placement during labour decreases the likelihood of requiring general anaesthesia for caesarean section.

9. Accept nothing less than a perfect block and complete pain relief during labour, since the epidural may be needed for caesarean section later on.

10. Have two experienced anaesthesiologists available when general anaesthesia is required. Take all steps of aspiration prophylaxis.

11. If general anaesthesia cannot be avoided and there is anticipated difficult airway, it is safe to do an "awake intubation" with a fibreoptic scope. Be prepared for failed tracheal intubation.

12. Administer 100% oxygen during regional anaesthesia until the newborn is delivered and the quality of block is ensured.

13. Aggressive chest physiotherapy, oxygen supplementation and nursing in semirecumbent position improve patient's respiratory status in the postoperative period.

Chapter 19

Neurological Diseases and Anaesthesia

A pregnant patient with neurological disease poses a challenge to the anaesthesiologist. Common problems encountered are Epilepsy and Spinal Cord Injury.

EPILEPSY

Epilepsy found in approximately 0.5% of parturients; the frequency of seizures does not change with pregnancy but can increase due to sleep deprivation, irregular drug therapy, eclampsia, metabolic, toxic or infective conditions. They may have their first seizure during pregnancy or may have seizures only during pregnancy.

Isolated seizures usually do not have deleterious effect on the foetus but injury to the mother and intra-uterine deaths are known to occur.

Status epilepticus can result in foetal and maternal death; immediate management includes protection of the airway, left uterine displacement and anticonvulsants like diazepam or thiopental.

Epileptic patients can have a safe pregnancy, though the incidence of complications such as pre-eclampsia, bleeding and premature labour is more.

They can have a normal vaginal delivery though the chances of obstetric intervention and caesarean section are more.

An epileptic seizure can occur during labour or within 24 hours of delivery; when it occurs during labour, there is foetal bradycardia. A postictal parturient may require immediate caesarean section.

Management

- Epileptic patients desirous of pregnancy can have their antiepileptic drugs (AEDs) withdrawn if they are seizure-free. If this is not possible, then lowest effective dose of single drug is recommended.
- Commonly used drugs include phenytoin, phenobarbital, valproate and carbamazepine. Except for trimethadione, which is contraindicated during pregnancy, other AED have not been consistently proven to be teratogenic.
- Two newer AEDs, Gabapentin and Lamotrigine do not appear to be teratogenic in animals.
- Serum levels of AEDs should be assessed every month during pregnancy; every week during last month of pregnancy and at the onset of labour. The doses must be readjusted during the postpartum period to avoid toxicity.

Anaesthetic Considerations

Pethidine and Phenothiazines are avoided in an epileptic patient; seizures are noted after pethidine administration, attributed to its metabolite norpethidine. Phenothiazines lower the seizure threshold.

Nitrous oxide appears to be safe during labour.

Epidural anaesthesia is safe during labour, delivery and caesarean section.

Low blood concentration of local anaesthetics seen after epidural block, act as anticonvulsants.

Spinal anaesthesia is safe but seizures can occur.

Caffine, used to treat post-dural puncture headache can cause postpartum seizure.

General Anaesthesia

Methohexital, Ketamine and Propofol have been associated with seizure like activity.

Anticonvulsants must be continued during fasting period.

General anaesthesia is induced with thiopental, succinylcholine and maintained with oxygen, nitrous oxide and isoflurane. If non-depolarising muscle relaxants are needed, Atracurium is used.

Avoid pethidine for postoperative analgesia.

SPINAL CORD INJURY

Spinal cord injury (SCI) in women of child bearing age occurs due to trauma, infection and neoplasia. The anaesthesiologist can be called upon to manage a pregnant patient with acute SCI or may face a pregnant patient with chronic SCI presenting for delivery.

Acute Spinal Cord Injury

- Assess the airway and breathing
- Stabilise the cervical spine
- Assess circulation.

Obstetric consultation to evaluate condition of the foetus, manage pre-term labour, assess need for urgent caesarean section:

1. In foetal distress
2. Foetus is of viable gestation age but survival of the mother is in doubt.

Foetal monitoring in third trimester is a must as it provides information about maternal perfusion and foetal well-being. There is loss of thermoregulation below the level of injury; it can lead to hypothermia in the patient.

Respiratory compromise may be exacerbated by changes due to pregnancy; the degree of compromise can be assessed by use of spirometry and blood gas analysis. Chest physiotherapy should be instituted early.

Hypotension may present due to neurogenic shock, hypovolaemia and bradycardia (due to damage to cardiac accelerator fibres). Usual signs of intraperitoneal haemorrhage may be obscured by SCI, gravid uterus and increased blood volume of pregnancy. It is corrected by fluid administration (monitor heart rate, urine output and CVP) with emphasis on left uterine displacement.

Consider ionotropes (dopamine, dobutamine) in low doses. They may lower placental blood flow hence foetal monitoring is essential.

Bradycardia (can occur during suction and intubation) is treated by use of atropine.

High dose of IV methylprednisolone within 8 hours of SCI may improve neurological outcome. Loading dose 30 mg/kg slow bolus followed by infusion of 5.4 mg/kg/hour over 24 hours. Monitor blood sugar especially in diabetics.

Adjuvant therapy: Ryle's tube, urinary catheter, pressure area relief every 2 hours, H_2 receptor antagonist for prophylaxis against stress ulcers.

Thromboembolic prophylaxis
Intermittent calf muscle compression
Compression stocking
Low molecular weight heparin.

Neurological shock usually lasts for 1 to 3 weeks; during this period if the level of SCI is above T 10 and complete transection has occurred, surgery can be done without anaesthesia but this is debatable. Transition phase may be difficult to define and risk of autonomic hyper-reflexia may exist.

Chronic Spinal Cord Injury

Patients with spinal cord injury frequently experience:
• Urinary tract infections
• Anaemia
• Disuse muscle atrophy
• Bedsores
• DVT and thromboembolic events.

With high-level spinal cord injuries (above T 5) parturient are at risk of:

- Postural hypotension
- Pneumonitis due to failure to cough out secretions
- Respiratory failure
- Autonomic hyper-reflexia (AH).

Autonomic hyper-reflexia may be triggered by urinary retention, constipation, uterine contraction and surgical stimulus.

It often occurs at the onset of labour but can occur in antepartum, intrapartum and postpartum periods.

Autonomic hyper-reflexia is characterised by hypertension, headache, anxiety, sweating, bradycardia, increased spasticity and cutaneous vasodilatation above the level of the lesion.

Management

If the risk of autonomic hyper-reflexia is low (lesion below T 7, with no history of autonomic hyper-reflexia), an IV line with regular NIBP measurement will suffice; systemic analgesics may be given to these patients.

If symptoms of AH appear or the risk is high from the outset:

- An epidural catheter is inserted.
- Invasive BP monitoring is done.
- Continuous ECG monitoring.
- Monitoring of uterine contractions.
- Continuous foetal monitoring.
- Pulse oximetry is used.

- Mechanical support of ventilation may be needed.
- Systemic analgesics are avoided for the fear of respiratory depression.

Regional anaesthesia techniques control hypertensive response of AH and prevent mass motor response.

Spinal or epidural anaesthesia can be used for labour and caesarean section. Continuous epidural block by maintaining a constant level of block is the best.

The epidural should be placed before the onset of labour and it should be left in place for 48 hours post-delivery.

Bupivacaine in low concentration or even .5% can be used for labour analgesia; pethidine can be added to local anaesthetic infusion to minimise the dose of LA and loss of sympathetic tone.

Spinal is more effective in preventing AH than epidural and is the technique of choice in patients requiring surgery, who are at risk of AH. It is recommended for emergency caesarean section.

For elective Caesarean section, CSE technique is best.

General anaesthesia is needed when RA is not possible.

Gastric emptying is delayed in patients having high SCI; full aspiration prophylaxis is needed.

Blood loss is poorly tolerated; must be diligently replaced.

Pressure areas should be carefully padded.

Hypothermia should be prevented.

Full monitoring along with temperature and invasive blood pressure monitoring is done.

These patients should be adequately hydrated.

Airway management can be difficult because of airway oedema and cervical spine disease.

Premedication with nifedepine and use of anti-hypertensive drug in addition to General anaesthesia may be necessary in patients at risk of AH. Low doses of induction agents are needed.

Scoline avoided for a period beginning 3days after SCI till 9 months.

Isoflurane is the drug of choice because of direct depression of peripheral vascular tone with minimal negative inotropy and arrhythmogenic action.

Tracheal extubation is considered only when patient is warm, stable, awake with no residual neuromuscular blockade.

Respiratory insufficiency may require postoperative ventilation.

Chapter 20

Anaesthesia for Kyphoscoliotic Parturient

Kyphoscoliosis is a rotational deformity of spine and ribs. It may be either primary (idiopathic) or secondary to neuromuscular or connective tissue disorders. Impairment of cardiorespiratory system occurs depending upon the level of spine and severity of curvature deformity. Severe scoliosis results in:

- Reduced lung volumes
- V/Q mismatch
- Reduced response to carbon dioxide
- Increased pulmonary vascular resistance
- Impaired cardiorespiratory reserve.

The majority of maternal deaths are due to cardio-respiratory failure, while obstetric complications account for relatively few.

Problems in Kyphoscoliotic Patients

- *Increased oxygen demand*: In kyphoscoliotic patient with restrictive pattern, rise in tidal volume is not possible and increase in minute ventilation is achieved by increasing the respiratory rate, resulting in increased work of breathing. Oxygen consumption increases by 40% in the first stage and by 70% in the second stage of labour.

- Diaphragm is entirely responsible for increasing minute ventilation; as uterus enlarges into the abdominal cavity in midgestation, it hampers the diaphragmatic movement leading to decreased FRC (functional residual capacity) and CC (closing capacity) resulting in ventilation-perfusion mismatch and reduced arterial oxygen content.

- Upper airway resistance rises during pregnancy because of mucosal hyperaemia and increased secretions. These changes result in snoring and obstructive sleep apnoea.

- In kyphoscoliosis, there is an increased peripheral vascular resistance; increased cardiac output that occurs in pregnancy can precipitate right heart failure. Pulmonary hypertension, not responding to oxygen therapy, carries a grave maternal prognosis and is an indication for termination of pregnancy. Death during labour or in early postpartum period is common with pulmonary hypertension.

- Complications are more likely in older parturients with severe kyphoscoliosis or with underlying neuromuscular disease. Others at risk are primipara who develop fatigue during prolonged labour. Premature labour is more common.

Anaesthetic Management

All types of anaesthesia have been tried and can be technically difficult to administer.

Antepartum maternal assessment focuses on:

- Cardiorespiratory status both current as well as past.
- Presence of coexisting disease.
- Prognosis of associated neuromuscular disorders. In patients with scoliosis resulting from neuromuscular disorders, anaesthetic considerations specific to those disorders should be reviewed.

- If respiratory compromise is evident, respiratory evaluation with special attention to the presence of dyspnoea, tachypnoea, exercise tolerance and pulmonary function is carried out.
- In patients with a known cardiac disease or in patients with curves greater than 60°, cardiologic evaluation to assess ventricular size and function and pulmonary vascular pressures is done.
- Admission to the hospital for the last weeks of the pregnancy enhances the likelihood that maternal decompensation will be recognised early and morbidity and mortality prevented.
- Oxygen therapy intermittently during the day, and continuously overnight may improve the maternal condition and reduce foetal risk.

Epidural anaesthesia with local anaesthetic alone or with a local anaesthetic-opioid mixture can be given.

In parturients with significant cardiovascular compromise, a dilute local anaesthetic and opioid mixture (bupivacaine 0.0625 to 0.125% with 2-4 mg/ml fentanyl at infusion rates of 8 to 15 ml/hr) provides excellent first stage and good second stage analgesia with fewer haemodynamic consequences compared with more concentrated local anaesthetic solution.

Combined spinal epidural (CSE) analgesia with intrathecal opioids can also be given for labour analgesia.

The goals in the anaesthetic management of parturients with pulmonary hypertension include:

1. Avoid pain, hypertension, hypoxaemia, hypercarbia and acidosis, because these increase pulmonary vascular resistance (PVR).
2. Avoid myocardial depression because cardiac output will be further decreased.
3. Maintenance of intravascular volume and preload.
4. Maintenance of systemic vascular resistance so as to ensure myocardial perfusion and prevent right to left shunting.

Systemic hypotension resulting from regional block may lead to right ventricular ischaemia and profound decrease in cardiac output. Because cardiac output is relatively fixed in patients with pulmonary hypertension, hypotension due to decreased systemic vascular resistance may elicit little effective physiologic compensation and may be difficult to treat pharmacologically.

Alternatives to regional block include patient controlled intravenous analgesia (PCA) with parenteral analgesics (fentanyl, meperidine) and inhalation of a 50:50 mixture of oxygen and nitrous oxide.

General anaesthesia may be preferable because it provides airway and ventilatory control. Unless there are technical difficulties or maternal decompensation is imminent, there is a role for regional anaesthesia. A slow incremental extension of an epidural or a subarachnoid block provides ideal conditions for operative delivery and postoperative analgesia.

Particular attention should be paid to the dose of local anaesthetic because the patient's small size renders usual volumes toxic.

In patients with severe curves, subarachnoid hyperbaric local anaesthetic solution may pool in dependant portions of the spine, resulting in an inadequate block. Supplementing the block with isobaric formulations of local anaesthetics may improve the quality of the block.

General anaesthesia may be used because of:

- Maternal preference
- Maternal cardiopulmonary disease
- Technical difficulties related to regional block.

Problems and Precautions for General Anaesthesia

1. Thorough evaluation of the maternal airway is necessary because scoliosis itself is associated with difficult laryngoscopy and intubation.
2. Many patients with scoliosis resulting from neuromuscular disease have pre-existing airway obstruction and may have sleep apnoea; these patients may be at particular risk for airway complications perioperatively.
3. Postoperatively, elements of laryngeal incompetence and impaired swallowing may further decrease the integrity of the airway defence mechanism.
4. Potential hazards of general anaesthesia in parturients with pulmonary hypertension include the increased pulmonary artery pressures during

laryngoscopy and intubation; reduced venous return due to positive pressure ventilation and negative inotropism of anaesthetic agents.

These adverse effects can be attenuated by an opioid supplemental induction and maintenance technique. Nitrous oxide should be avoided because it increases PVR.

These patients should be in an intensive care setting for up to a week following delivery because major cardiopulmonary complications are common during this period.

Anaesthesia, tracheal intubation, and surgery result in mucociliary dysfunction and abnormal or retrograde mucous flow. Reduced competence of the larynx increases the potential for post-extubation aspiration. Coughing and bucking, at the end of surgery may transiently and significantly reduce FRC, resulting in further ventilation/perfusion mismatch and hypoxaemia.

Criteria for postoperative extubation must include assessment of preoperative respiratory function.

An assessment of respiratory muscle strength and ability to support the airway should be made in all patients, but it is particularly important in patients with pre-existing compromise.

Other factors contributing to postoperative hypoxaemia in scoliotic parturients are:

Increased ventilation/perfusion mismatch,

Increased alveolar to arterial oxygen gradient,

Inhibition of hypoxic pulmonary vasoconstriction,

Decreased cardiac output,
Underlying pre-existent pulmonary disease,
Restriction of chest wall movement.

Important Tips

1. Both general and regional anaesthesia is suitable in mild scoliosis.
2. It is important to evaluate the patient and the cardio-respiratory reserve using:
   a. Patient's functional ability (both respiratory and cardiac).
   b. Respiratory spirometry.
   c. Arterial blood gas (ABG).
   d. Echocardiography.
3. These patients are often underweight, so the dosages need to be carefully titrated. Even a test dose of local anaesthetic may become more than the spinal dose, so needs to be modified accordingly.
4. Fluid replacement should be closely monitored.
5. Spinal anaesthesia may not be technically difficult but there is danger of very high or low levels block, making the technique, unpredictable.
6. General anaesthesia is difficult due to problems of airway control and ventilation abnormalities. When scoliosis is secondary to neuromuscular disorder, choosing the neuromuscular relaxant is difficult.

7. Residual neuromuscular blockade in presence of pre-existing muscle wasting may require post-operative ventilator support.

8. The patient with expected difficult intubation should preferably be intubated and extubated awake, paralyzed with titrated dose of neuro-muscular blocking agents, induced and sedated with careful titration of drugs.

9. Combined spinal epidural anaesthesia (CSE) with its merits of both spinal and epidural block may be preferred.

10. Accidental dural puncture while performing epidural may result in total spinal anaesthesia.

11. Anaesthetists may face problems in kyphoscoliotic spine while performing regional block. It may be technically difficult to place epidural catheter, as the depth of space may be unpredictable. Epidural space may be just at 2-3 cm depth.

12. Spread of local anaesthetics in spinal as well as epidural anaesthesia may be erratic.

13. The anaesthetic technique should be tailored to meet individual patient's needs, weighing the merits and demerits of available alternatives.

14. Choose a technique in which one is most confident.

15. Risk of respiratory failure persists in the post-operative period also.

Exemplary case in a 29 years old parturient with severely kyphoscoliotic spine (Figs 20.1 and 20.2). Caesarean delivery was successfully conducted under CSE. CSE was performed in sitting position with wide

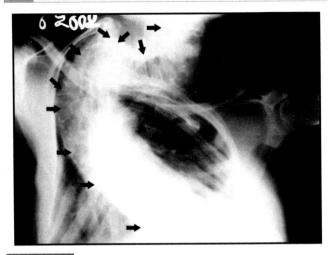

Figure 20.1

X-ray PA view showing kyphoscoliotic spine

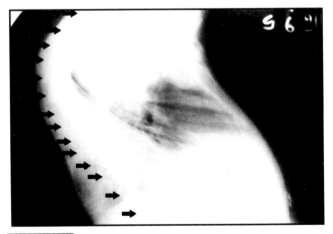

Figure 20.2

X-ray chest lateral view showing kyphosis

exposure of spine by leaving back of patient undraped to view the curvatures and have a better projection of spine. Epidural catheter was placed through 18G Tuohy's needle. Depth was just 3 cm and catheter was introduced 2 cm further. Test dose of xylocaine was reduced. Spinal was given one level below with paramedian approach with 6 mg bupivacaine 0.5% heavy. Table tilt was titrated to achieve sensory level of block up to T7-8 only as assessed by sharp pinprick of needle. Low level of spinal block was kept with fear of respiratory compromise and to maintain patient's coughing ability.

Preoperative evaluation and anticipation of problem is the key to success in all difficult cases. Low dose sequential combined spinal and epidural block not only provides satisfactory surgical conditions and post-operative analgesia, but also the risk coverage of failure of one component of technique over the other in the back of mind of anaesthesiologist.

Chapter 21

HIV, Anaesthesia and Anaesthetist

Worldwide, 50 million people are infected with the human immunodeficiency virus (HIV), and 43% are women. Perinatal vertical transmission of HIV accounts for most new paediatric cases. Elective caesarean delivery combined with antiretroviral therapy perioperatively and abandonment of breastfeeding postoperatively reduces vertical HIV transmission. The majority of these females being in reproductive age group, come for obstetrical care. This group of females requires special attention regarding perinatal transmission and the implications of infection with regard to pregnancy.

CENTRE FOR DISEASE CONTROL (CDC) CLASSIFICATION OF HIV

Group I: Acute infection

Group II: Asymptomatic infection

Group III: Persistent generalised lymphadenopathy

Group IV: Sub-grouping as follows:
a. Constitutional disease
b. Neurological disease
c. Secondary infection
d. Secondary neoplasm
e. Other conditions

Key Points

1. *Type of anaesthesia*: General anaesthesia can be given to these patients; GA leads to immunosuppresion within 15 minutes of induction, which lasts for 3-11days. Coexistent hepatobiliary disease or nephropathy of AIDS may alter pharmacokinetics and pharmacodynamics of anaesthetic drugs.

2. *Safety of regional anaesthesia*: Infection with HIV in pregnancy often raises questions about the safety of regional anaesthesia in these patients. It has been suggested that the introduction of a spinal needle in an HIV infected parturient would spread the disease into the CNS, leading to the development of neurological sequelae. Nevertheless, recent analysis of the problem has shown HIV infection should not contraindicate use of regional anaesthesia.

3. *Implications of antiviral drugs*: Consider implications of antiviral anti-microbial therapy. Metabolism of following drugs is decreased in presence of protease inhibitors.
   - Fentanyl
   - Pethidine
   - Midazolam
   - Diazepam.

4. *Treatment of complications*: The parturients are at risk of developing postoperative complications such as wound healing impairment, bronchitis and pneumonia requiring prolonged antibiotic therapy depending upon their immune status.

5. *Mode of transmission:*
   - Rectal or vaginal intercourse
   - Blood product transfusion
   - Shared intravenous needles
   - Vertical transmission
   - Occupational acquisition.

6. *Risk of occupational infection*: Risk of anaesthetist contracting infection from HIV infected patient is 0.001-0.129% per year.

The occupational exposure of a health care worker (HCW)
due to contact with a known HIV patient can result from:
- Percutaneous inoculation
- Contamination of an open wound
- Contamination of breached skin
- Contamination of mucous membranes including
  conjunctiva.
7. Universal precautions taken while handling HIV + patients
   - Effective hand washing (Fig. 21.1)
   - Double gloving (special puncture resistant glove if
     available)
   - No-touch technique
   - Using eye glasses, eye protection shield, disposable masks,
     impermeable gowns and boots.
8. Personnel attending the patient in the operating room should
   remove all protective gown, gloves, eye-shields, etc. before
   leaving the operation theatre.
9. Cleaning of anaesthetic equipment:
   - Inactivation of the HIV. Heat and chemical disinfectants
     like sodium hypochlorite, glutaraldehyde and methyl, ethyl
     and isopropyl alcohol are effective
   - Contaminated area should be covered with 1 % sodium
     hypochlorite solution for 10 min, mopped up and cleaned
     with a neutral detergent solution
   - Anaesthetic machine. On work surfaces, use disposable
     impervious covers or trays that can be sterilized or
     disposed off
   - Laryngoscopes blades—clean with warm soap and water,
     then autoclave or soak in 1% hypochlorite solution or
     70% alcohol for 20 min, rinse with distilled water and dry
   - Breathing systems/airway devices. Use disposable
     breathing systems as far as possible. Place filter between
     absorber and disposable circuits and also between
     ventilators. Use disposable tracheal tubes, airways
   - Disposal items such as gloves, syringes, etc. should be
     shredded, cut or mutilated before disposal followed by

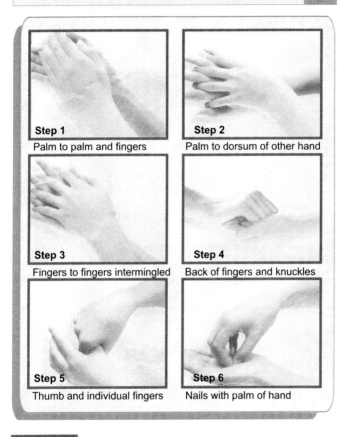

Step 1
Palm to palm and fingers

Step 2
Palm to dorsum of other hand

Step 3
Fingers to fingers intermingled

Step 4
Back of fingers and knuckles

Step 5
Thumb and individual fingers

Step 6
Nails with palm of hand

Figure 21.1

Hand washing and disinfection

deep burial or properly accounted for before disposal. Liquid wastes should be treated with a chemical disinfectant for decontamination, neutralised and flushed into sewer.

10. *Packing, storage and transport of wastes:* All segregated and disinfected waste should be placed in proper containers; all

containers used for storage should be provided with a proper lid and labelled. The containers should be inaccessible to scavengers and protected from insects, birds animals and rain. The sharp waste after pre-treatment should be broken before placing in the container. The waste should be transported in vehicles authorised for this purpose only. Waste should not be stored in the place where it is generated for a period of more than two days.

11. *Management of needle stick injuries*: Acquisition of HIV from occupational exposure via a needle stick injury is a dreaded complication. Transmission of HIV after a needle-stick injury is 0.3% versus 6-37% for hepatitis B in a non-immune health worker and 2% for percutaneous exposure to hepatitis C. Suture needles are the most common sources of injury in operating and delivery rooms. The volume transmitted depends on the depth of penetration and also whether it is a hollow bored needle or suture needle.

12. *The types of exposure are (Fig. 21.2)*:
    1. Percutaneous—needle-stick or cut by a sharp instrument.
    2. Mucous membranes—eyes, mouth, nose.
    3. Direct contact with non-intact skin for more than 1 minute in cases of dermatitis, eczema, laceration or an open wound.

13. The other sources of HIV transmission in health co-workers are semen, vaginal secretions, synovial, peritoneal, pleural, pericardial, cerebrospinal and amniotic fluids.

14. Urine, saliva or faeces are not sources unless contaminated with blood.

15. *Post-exposure prophylaxis (Fig. 21.3)*:
    • All health care workers (HCWs) working in institutions should be provided with a detailed protocol to be followed.
        • *Step 1*: Determine exposure code. All such HCWs should be classified according to the exposure code,
        • *Step 2*: Determine the HIV status code and
        • *Step 3*: Follow the standard recommendations given below
            • Use of multidrug, prophylactic, antiviral therapy for HIV exposure is now recommended.

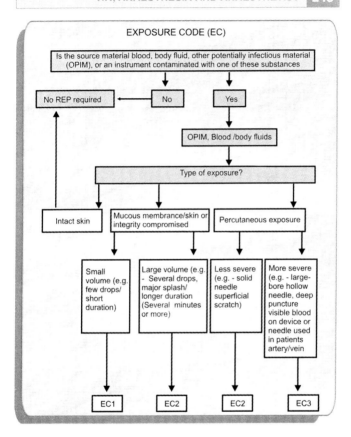

Figure 21.2

HIV exposure code

- New antiretroviral drugs
  1. Nucleoside analogogue reverse transcriptase inhibitors
  2. Non-nucleoside analogues reverse transcriptase inhibitors
  3. Protease inhibitors.

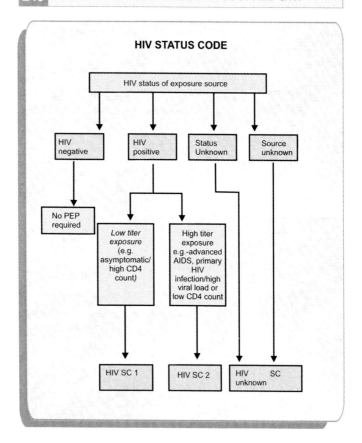

Figure 21.3

HIV status code: The main purpose of determining HIV status code is to know the HIV status of source of exposure. It may be classified into three categories: HIV SC1, HIV SC2, HIV SC unknown

Step 1 (Exposure code)

Exposure code	Route status	Volume of potential infected material
EC 1	Integrity of skin/mucous membrane compromised	Small
EC 2	Integrity of skin/mucous membrane compromised	Large
	Percutaneous exposure	Small (superficial scratch, solid needle)
EC 3	Percutaneous exposure	Severe (hollow) needle, deep puncture, clear cut exposure of blood
No post-exposure prophylaxis	Intact skin	Irrespective

Step 2 (HIV status code)

Test status	Infectivity	Status code	Recommendations
HIV negative	No risk		No need of prophylaxis

Contd...

Test status	Infectivity	Status code	Recommendations
HIV positive	Low titer exposure (asymptomatic) high CD4 count,	HIV SC 1	As per exposure See recommendation table
HIV positive	Higher titer exposure (AIDS, high or increasing viral load, low CD4 count)	HIV SC 2	As per exposure See recommendation table
HIV status unknown	—	HIV SC unknown	If the circumstances suggest risk, EC code is 2 or 3, consider basic regimen
HIV source unknown	—	HIV SC unknown	If the circumstances suggest risk, EC code is 2 or 3, consider basic regimen

Recommendations for Post-exposure Prophylaxis

Exposure code	HIV status code	Recommendations
1	1	Risk is low and Prophylaxis is not warranted. Whether risk outweighs the drug toxicity should be decided by treating physician
1	2	Consider basic regimen Zidovudine 500 in two to three divided doses + Lamivudine 150 mg twice daily for four weeks
2	1	Recommend basic regimen
2	2	Recommend expanded regimen Zidovudine 500 in two to three divided doses + Lamivudine 150 mg twice daily + indinavir

Contd...

Contd...

Exposure code	HIV status code	Recommendations
		800 mg every 8 hrly or Nelfinvir 750 mg three times a day
3	1 or 2	Recommend expanded regimen
2 or 3	Unknown	Consider depending upon the netting, if suggests risk, basic regimen is recommended

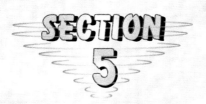

SECTION
5

CRITICAL CARE IN
OBSTETRICS

Chapter 22

Arterial Blood Gas Analysis

The maintenance of normal acid-base balance in the blood is a vital homeostatic function of the body. Any significant change in the H^+ ion concentration is incompatible with life and often occurs in patients who are critically ill. Not uncommonly, the realisation that deterioration is related to a change in the acid-base status of the patient dawns too late, which is why a sharp clinical acumen, grasp of underlying physiology and correct interpretation of laboratory data is very important.

Physiology

Acid is being continually produced in the body through metabolic processes. Despite this addition of acids to the body, the pH is maintained within a narrow range of 7.35-7.45.

Acidosis = Increased acid or decreased alkali.

Alkalosis = Increased alkali or decreased acid.

Metabolic disorders = Primary change is in HCO_3.

Respiratory disorders = Primary change is in $PaCO_2$

The pH is maintained by two major mechanisms: Compensation and Correction

Compensation: Alters the component not primarily responsible for abnormality. It tries to bring the values towards normal but is never complete.

Correction: pH is normalised by altering the component that is primarily responsible for the abnormality. It may be acute or chronic.

Immediate large scale change in pH is prevented by buffers which include HCO_3, phosphates and protein buffers.

Regulation of pH ultimately depends on lungs and the kidneys. Role of the lungs is to eliminate CO_2 which is the principal end product of acid metabolism in response to changes in blood pH. Role of the kidneys is to retain HCO_3^- and eliminate H^+ ions of nonvolatile acids.

For every 10 mm Hg rise or fall in $PaCO_2$ from the normal (40 mm Hg), there is a change in pH by .08 units in the opposite direction (e.g. for a 20 mm Hg rise in $PaCO_2$, pH will fall by 20 × .08 =.16, therefore pH=7.4 – .16=7.24)

A 7-7.5 mEq /L change in HCO_3^- level, changes the pH by .1 units in the same direction.

Normal Blood Gas Values during Pregnancy

PaO_2	104-108 (same as non-pregnant patient)
$PaCO_2$	27-32 (non-pregnant value 38-45)
HCO_3^-	18-31 (non-pregnant value 24-31)
pH	7.4-7.5 (non-pregnant value 7.36-7.44)

Base Excess (BE)

It is a measure of metabolic acid level and is useful in diagnosis of metabolic disorders. Normal values are normally zero $\pm$ 2.

Positive values indicate metabolic alkalosis; negative values metabolic acidosis.

BE may be used to estimate the amount of treatment (neutralisation) required to overcome the metabolic acidosis (or alkalosis).

To correct metabolic acidosis, following amount of $NaHCO_3$ is suggested:

$NaHCO_3$ dose (mmol) = BE (mmol/lit) × Body weight (kg) ÷ 3
(8.4% $NaHCO_3$ solution contains 1 mmol $NaHCO_3$ per ml)

or

$NaHCO_3$ deficit = .5 × Body weight (kg) × (desired HCO_3 – actual serum HCO_3)

This is the total dose needed to correct metabolic acidosis; it should be given in small doses of $NaHCO_3$ (50-100 mL) at a time; repeatedly assess BE and pH.

Or: Give half the dose as IV bolus and the remaining as an infusion over 4-6 hours.

Or: Administer $NaHCO_3$ at a frequency and dose to keep the arterial pH above 7.3.

Sodium bicarbonate therapy is considered harmful because:

• It leads to an increase in carbon dioxide load and more acidosis if there is inadequate wash out by the lungs.

• Severe myocardial depression has been reported in cases of heart failure and patients of ischaemic heart disease.

• It causes hyperosmolarity, hypernatraemia and hypokalaemia.

ANION GAP

It is an acid-base parameter that is used to determine whether the metabolic acidosis is due to accumulation of H^+ ions or due to loss of HCO_3^- ions.

$$\text{Anion gap} = Na^+ - Cl^- - HCO_3^-$$
$$\text{Normal anion gap} = 12 \, (\pm 4) \, mEq/L$$

A clue to mixed acid-base disorder, is the anion gap (AG) and HCO_3 relationship:

Change in anion gap above 12 is called $\Delta AG = (AG - 12)$

Change of HCO_3 below 24 is called $\Delta HCO_3 = (24 - HCO_3)$

$\Delta AG/\Delta HCO_3$ is called gap – gap

For simple anion gap acidosis, gap – gap = 1

Hyperchloraemic acidosis gap – gap = 0

Metabolic acidosis with metabolic alkalosis gap – gap ≥ 1.5.

Uteroplacental Effects of Acid-base Balance

Acid-base imbalance affects the foetus directly (through placental transmission) and indirectly (by changes in placental perfusion).

Changes in maternal PCO_2 result in rapid changes in foetal PCO_2 in the same direction because CO_2 diffuses rapidly across placenta.

Changes in HCO_3^- and H^+ are much slow; maternal metabolic acidosis and alkalosis will cause little change in foetal pH over several hours.

The effect of acidosis on placental circulation is vaso-dilation but this is opposed by sympathoadrenal stimulation, resulting in very little change in uterine blood flow.

Maternal alkalosis (respiratory more than metabolic), results in vasoconstriction of uterine vessels and reduction in uteroplacental blood flow.

Alkalosis causes the maternal oxyhaemoglobin dissociation curve to shift to left, thus reducing the amount of available oxygen to the foetus.

The combination of vasoconstriction and reduced oxygen delivery in severe alkalosis (pH > 7.65) will cause foetal hypoxaemia and metabolic acidosis.

In milder respiratory alkalosis (as in labour), placental perfusion is maintained and maternal and foetal PCO_2 equilibrate across the placenta. This increases foetal pH, shifts foetal oxyhaemoglobin dissociation curve to left increasing oxygen uptake and resulting in higher foetal oxygen saturation.

Clinical Situations in which ABG Analysis is Useful

- Respiratory disorders
- Hypoxaemic respiratory failure
- Degree of hypoxia
- Effect of therapy
- Hypercapnic respiratory failure
- Need for mechanical ventilation
- Effect of mechanical ventilation
- Shock
- Sepsis
- DIC
- Renal failure
- Poisonings.

TREATMENT OF ACID-BASE DISORDERS

Respiratory Conditions

1. Diagnose

2. Treat the underlying disease
3. Supportive therapy
   - Bronchodilators
   - Analgesia for pain relief
   - Mechanical ventilation.

Metabolic Acidosis

1. Treat the underlying cause rather than empirical treatment with sodabicarbonate.
2. Empirical treatment is indicated when pH is very low to cause fatal arrhythmias and hypotension.

Consider Sodium Bicarbonate Therapy In:

1. Severe metabolic acidosis with pH less than 7.10
2. BE-ECF less than -15 mmol/L
3. Metabolic acidosis is accompanied with hyperkalaemia or in cases of renal failure.

Metabolic Alkalosis

1. Find and treat the underlying cause.
2. Usual causes are diuretic therapy, excessive vomiting, diarrhoea, gut fistulas, etc.
3. Treatment of underlying pathology and normal saline fluid administration resolves most of the cases.
4. Rarely development of contraction alkalosis may require administration vitamin C in drip or acid infusion.
5. Diamox tablet (Acetazolamide), a carbonic dehydrogenase inhibitor given orally for few days may help to restore normal blood pH.

Arterial Blood Gas Analysis

Normal Values

pH 7.35 to 7.45

PaO_2 80-100 mm Hg

O_2 saturation > 95%

PCO_2 35 to 45 mm Hg HCO_3 22 to 26 mEq/L

BE – 2 to + 2 mmol/L

AG 12 ± 2 mmol/L.

Assessment of Arterial Oxygenation

1. Assess the arterial O_2 saturation (95-100%) by pulse oximetry

2. Assess the PO_2 (80-100 mmHg)

    As a rule of thumb, % of inspired O_2 × 5 = Predicted minimum PaO_2.

$PaCO_2$—pH Relationship in Respiratory Acid-base Balance

- For every acute rise of $PaCO_2$ by 10 mm Hg, pH decreased by 0.07 unit

- For every acute fall of $PaCO_2$ by 10 mm Hg, pH increased by 0.08 unit.

$PaCO_2$—HCO_3 Relationship in Respiratory Acid-base Balance

- For every acute rise of $PaCO_2$ by 10 mm Hg, HCO_3 increases by 1 mmol/lt

- For every chronic rise of $PaCO_2$ by 10 mm Hg, HCO_3 increases by 4 mmol/lt
- For every acute fall of $PaCO_2$ by 10 mm Hg, HCO_3 decreases by 2 mmol/lt
- For every chronic fall of $PaCO_2$ by 10 mm Hg, HCO_3 decreases by 6 mmol/lt.

SUMMARY OF ACID-BASE DISORDERS

ABG disorder	Primary disorder	Compensatory response	Expected compensation
Metabolic acidosis	Decreased HCO_3	Decreased PCO_2	$PaCO_2 = (1.5 \times$ serum $HCO_3) + 8$
Metabolic alkalosis	Increased HCO_3	Increased PCO_2	$PaCO_2 = (0.7 \times$ serum $HCO_3) + 20$
Respiratory acidosis	Increased PCO_2	Increased HCO_3	Acute: pH $= .08 \times \dfrac{(PaCO_2 - 40)}{10}$ Chronic: pH $= .03 \times \dfrac{(PaCO_2 - 40)}{10}$
Respiratory alkalosis	Decreased PCO_2	Decreased HCO_3	Acute: pH $= .08 \times \dfrac{(40 - PaCO_2)}{10}$ Chronic: pH $= .03 \times \dfrac{(40 - PaCO_2)}{10}$

pH, PCO_2 and HCO_3 Findings in Respiratory Acid-base Disorders

Nomenclature	pH	PCO_2	HCO_3
Respiratory acidosis Uncompensated (acute)	Low	Increased	Normal
Partly compensated (subacute)	Low	Increased	Increased
Compensated (chronic)	Normal	Increased	Increased
Respiratory alkalosis			
Uncompensated (acute)	Increased	Decreased	Normal
Partly compensated (subacute)	Increased	Decreased	Decreased
Compensated (chronic)	Normal	Decreased	Decreased

pH, PCO$_2$ and HCO$_3$ Findings in Metabolic Acid-base Disorders

Nomenclature	pH	PCO$_2$	HCO$_3$
Metabolic acidosis			
Uncompensated (acute)	Decreased	Normal	Decreased
Partly compensated (subacute)	Decreased	Decreased	Decreased
Compensated (chronic)	Normal	Decreased	Decreased
Metabolic alkalosis			
Uncompensated (acute)	Increased	Normal	Increased
Partly compensated (subacute)	Increased	Increased	Increased
Compensated (chronic)	Normal	Increased	Increased

Arterial Oxygen Tensions-Oxyhaemoglobin Saturation Relationship

	PaO$_2$ (mmHg)	SaO$_2$ (%)
Normal	97	97
Normal range	> 80	> 95
Hypoxaemia	< 80	< 95
Mild hypoxaemia	60-79	90-94
Moderate hypoxaemia	40-59	75-89
Severe hypoxaemia	< 40	< 75

Two major exceptions to the normal range of PaO_2 values shown above are: First, the newborn infant has a PaO_2 between 40-70 mm Hg. Second, oxygen tension values decrease with age. The general guideline is to subtract 1 mm Hg from the minimal 80 mm Hg level for every year over 60 years. This is not applicable to persons more than 90 years of age.

FiO_2-PaO_2 Relationship

FiO_2	Inspired oxygen (%)	PaO_2 (mm Hg)
0.21	21	> 100
0.4	40	> 200
0.5	50	I > 250
0.8	80	> 400
1.0	100	> 500

As a rule of thumb, % of inspired $O_2 \times 5$ = Predicted minimum PaO_2.

The ratio PaO_2:FiO_2 gives an idea of the degree of lung dysfunction:

PaO_2/FiO_2 ratio (for air) $= 105/.21 = 500$

    > 500 = Normal

    300-500 = Some degree of oxygenation problem

    200-300 = Acute lung injury

    < 200 = ARDS

Metabolic Acidosis: Approach to Differential Diagnosis

	Metabolic Acidosis	$\downarrow pH$ $\downarrow PCO_2$ $\downarrow HCO_3$	Anion gap 12 (± 4)
Raised anion gap		*Normal anion gap*	
	Loss of HCO_3	*Increased chlorides*	

Increased acid production	Decreased acid excretion	GIT	Renal	NH_4CL
1. Ketoaci- dosis (DM, Alcohol, Starvation)	1. Acute renal failure	1 Diarrhoea	1. Renal tubular acidosis	Poisoning and amino acids
2. Lactic acidosis	2. Chronic renal failure	2 Villous adenoma	2. Addison's disease	
3. Poisoning (Methanol, ethylene glycol)		3 Urinary diversion procedure		

SEVEN STEPS TO SUCCESSFUL AND RAPID ABG ANALYSIS

Step 1: Look at pH
Less than 7.35 (acidaemia)
More than 7.45 (alkalaemia)

Step 2: Look at PCO_2 and HCO_3
PCO_2 more than 45 mm Hg   Respiratory acidosis
PCO_2 less than 35 mm Hg   Respiratory alkalosis

HCO_3 less than 20 mmol/l   Metabolic acidosis
HCO_3 more than 28 mmol/l   Metabolic alkalosis

Step 3:

In primary respiratory disturbance, expect
Rise/Fall in pH = 0.08 × Rise/Fall in PCO_2
Yes   Acute change
No   Chronic change

Step 4:

If non-acute look for compensation
1. Respiratory acidosis
   • 6 to 24 hours
     Rise in HCO_3 = 1/10 × rise in PCO_2
   • 1 to 4 days
     Rise in HCO_3 = 4/10 × rise in PCO_2

2. Respiratory alkalosis
   • 1 to 2 hours
     Fall in HCO_3 = 2/10 × fall in PCO_2
   • More than 2 days
     Fall in HCO_3 = 5/10 × fall in PCO_2

   If change in HCO_3 is not as expected, then there is a superimposed primary metabolic disturbance
Or compensation is not complete.

Step 5:

If primary disturbance is metabolic and there is acidaemia: Is the anion gap increased? (Normal is 8-12)
i.e. $(Na^+) - (CL^-) - (HCO_3^-)$ is more than 14.

Step 6:

For metabolic disturbance, is there compensation?
Compensation in metabolic acidosis:
In metabolic acidosis:
Expected $PCO_2 = (1.5 \times HCO_3) + 8 \pm 2$

Compensation in metabolic alkalosis
Expected $PCO_2 = (0.7 \times HCO_3) + 21 \pm 1.5$

If respiratory compensation is not appropriate:

- Actual PCO_2 is more than expected—there is hidden primary respiratory acidosis.
- If actual PCO_2 is less than expected—then there is hidden primary respiratory alkalosis.

Step 7:

If there is increased anion gap acidosis, look for other metabolic disturbances by examining whether excess anion gap, i.e. measured HCO_3^+ (Anion GAP – 12) is 24 mmol/lit.

- In Absence of chronic respiratory acid-base disorder:
  If excess anion gap is less than 24, there is hidden non-gap acidosis.
  If excess anion gap is more than 24, there is co existing metabolic alkalosis along with metabolic acidosis.

Chapter 23

Critical Care in Obstetrics

The maternal morbidity and mortality is an indirect indicator of the quality of the obstetrics care. Advances in anaesthesia and critical care have improved the survival of critically sick patients. The management of obstetrical intensive care demands thorough understanding of the pregnancy induced physiological changes in the body organs and their functions. The overall incidence of admission of obstetritc patients to Intensive Care Unit is approximately 0.17% of deliveries. Common indications for admission to ICU are:

1. Worsening of preeclampsia.
2. Severe bleeding.
3. Maternal cardiac disease.
4. Pulmonary embolism.
5. Acute pulmonary oedema.
6. Hypovolaemic post-traumatic shock.

DIAGNOSTIC CRITERIA FOR SEVERE PREECLAMPSIA

BP > 160-180 mm Hg systolic or > 110 mm Hg diastolic
Proteinurea > 5 gm per 24 hours
Oligurea urine output < 500 ml per 24 hours
Cerebral or visual disturbances
Pulmonary oedema
Epigastric or right upper quadrant pain
Impaired liver functions
Thrombocytopenia
Elevated serum creatinine
Grand mal seizures
Foetal IUGR or oligohydramnios.

Eclampsia and Severe Preeclampsia

1. Patients with eclampsia and severe preeclampsia may need admission to Intensive Care Unit for control of their complications.

COMPLICATIONS OF SEVERE PREGNANCY INDUCED HYPERTENSION

Cardiovascular: Sever hypertension, pulmonary oedema
Renal: Oligurea, renal failure
Haematologic: Haemolysis, thrombocytopenia, DIC
Neurologic: Eclampsia, cerebral oedema, cerebral haemorrhage
Hepatic: Hepatocellular dysfunction, hepatic rupture
Uteroplacental: Abruption, IUGR, foetal distress, foetal death.

Management includes aggressive treatment of arterial blood pressure, complications and delivery of foetus.

Fluid management: Normal Saline or Ringer lactate, 100-125 ml/hour. Additional fluid volume of 1000-1500 ml may be needed prior to giving an epidural or vasodilator therapy to prevent an excessive fall in blood pressure. Close monitoring of fluid intake and output, haemodynamic parameters and clinical signs are necessary to prevent the onset of pulmonary oedema.

Antihypertensive therapy

• Arterial blood pressure should be controlled with antihypertensive drugs considered safe during pregnancy, sodium nitroprusside infusion and epidural blockade in difficult situations.

- Medical intervention is necessary when:
  Diastolic BP > 110 mm Hg
  Systolic BP > 160-180 mm Hg
  MAP > 140-150 mm Hg (increased risk of intra-cranial bleeding).

Drug	Action	Dosage	Comment
Hydralazine	Arterial vasodilator	5 mg IV; then 5-10 mg IV/20 min total of 40 mg; IV infusion 5-10 mg/hr titrated	Wait 20 min between doses. possible maternal hypotension
Labetalol	Selective alpha and non-selective beta blocker	20 mg IV, then 40-80 mg IV per 10 min to 300 mg total dose; IV infusion 1-2 mg/min, titrated	Less tachy-cardia and hypotension than hydra-lazine
Nifedipine	Ca^{++} channel blocker	10 mg by mouth; repeat after 30 min	Exaggerated effect if used with $MgSO_4$
Nitroglycerine	Relaxation of vascular smooth muscles	5 mcg/min infusion; double every 5 min	Continuous BP moni-toring; methemo-globinaemia
Sodium Nitroprusside	Vasodilator	.25 mcg/kg/min infusion; increase every 5 min	Continuous BP monitoring; potential cyanide toxicity

– Start with Hydralazine which will bring down the BP to 160-130 mm Hg. Systolic and 110-80 mm Hg diastolic in majority of cases.

– If 40 mg Hydralazine does not bring the BP down then proceed to use calcium channel blockers or labetalol.

– As a last resort use IV infusion of nitroglycerine or nitroprusside.

Control of Convulsions

• Magnesium sulphate may be used for prophylaxis and treatment of convulsions. The mechanism of action is probably vasodilatation and a central anticonvulsant effect. It has a wide margin of safety; therapeutic anticonvulsant serum magnesium levels are 4-6 mEq/L (5-8 mg/dl).

• Loading dose is 4 to 6 gm of $MgSO_4$ over 20 minutes followed by an infusion of 2-3 gm/hour for 24 hours. Another bolus of 2-4 gm may be repeated in case convulsions reoccur.

Side effects include prolonged effect of muscle relaxants, hypotension and oliguria. Urine output, patellar reflexes and respiratory rate should be monitored closely during $MgSO_4$ therapy. In presence of renal dysfunction, monitor serum magnesium levels.

• Whenever treating a patient with $MgSO_4$, patient must be observed for loss of tendon reflexes ($MgSO_4$

levels of 8 to 10 mEq/L), myocardial depression (MgSO$_4$ levels of 10-15 mEq/L), respiratory failure (MgSO$_4$ levels of 12-15 mEq/L) and cardiac arrest at 25-30 mEq/L.

- Treatment of severe MgSO$_4$ toxicity is discontinue the drug, administration of calcium gluconate, 10 ml of a 10% solution IV over 2 minutes (infusion of calcium gluconate may be needed under continuous cardiac monitoring) oxygen therapy and IPPR if necessary; diuretics (furosemide 20-40 mg, IV); stop calcium channel blockers, if in use.
- Convulsions can be terminated by a small dose of thiopentone sodium (50-100 mg) or diazepam (5-10 mg) while waiting for MgSO$_4$ to have its effect.
- Cerebral and visual disturbances often resolve spontaneously in few days after control of pre-eclampsia and delivery.
- HELLP syndrome and coagulation problems need close monitoring and management.
- Pulmonary oedema may require mechanical ventilation.

ANALGESIA AND ANAESTHESIA FOR PREECLAMPSIA

Regional blocks and general anaesthesia, both, are not without risk in presence of pregnancy induced hypertension.

Under regional anaesthesia, sympathetic blockade and peripheral vasodilatation can lead to hypotension and foetal distress in patients who are already volume contracted.

GA can result in significant systemic and pulmonary hypertension especially during endotracheal intubation and extubation.

Patients under regional blocks maintain stable systemic and pulmonary arterial pressures; there is a drop in mean arterial pressure, insignificant drop in systemic vascular resistance without change in cardiac index, peripheral vascular resistance and CVP; a significant increase in uterine blood flow is noted. Hypotension can be avoided by lateral maternal tilt, preloading with crystalloid solution and use of ephedrine.

Contraindications to RA include:

- Patient refusal
- Acute foetal distress requiring immediate delivery
- Local infection and septicaemia
- Spinal deformity
- Coagulopathy.

If preceded by volume loading, epidural anaesthesia appears beneficial and safe in severe preeclampsia.

A cautiously administered epidural is not only justified but the method of choice for anaesthesia in caesarean section or for labour analgesia, in patients with severe preeclampsia.

When GA is necessary, careful control of maternal blood pressure especially during induction and awakening, is essential.

PREECLAMPSIA MANAGEMENT PROTOCOL

1. ***Goals of therapy:***
   a. Control hypertension (BP > 180–160/110 mm Hg)
   b. Seizure prophylaxis/therapy
   c. Delivery of foetus and placenta
   d. Stabilization and correction of multisystem dysfunction

2. ***Management protocol***
   a. Control BP: Hydralazine 2.5 to 5 mg IV every 20 minutes to maintain BP < 160 mm Hg
   b. Seizure prophylaxis: $MgSO_4$ IV loading dose 4 to 6 gm over 20 minutes; maintenance dose of 2 to 3 gm/hour IV
   c. Delivery of foetus: induction of labour or caesarean section
   d. Stabilization/correction of multisystem dysfunction.

3. ***Clinical laboratory tests***
   Complete blood count, platelet count, serum creatinine, hepatic transaminase, lactic dehydrogenase, urine analysis. Additional tests: Fibrinogen, PT, PTT, uric acid and BUN, blood grouping and matching, 24 hour urine for protein and creatinine clearance.

4. ***Consultation***
   Obst/Gyn, Anaesthesiology, Neonatology.
   Depending on clinical situation: Critical care, Neurology, Nephrology.

Thromboembolic Disease and Pulmonary Embolism

Thromboembolic Disease (TED) in pregnancy is a leading cause of maternal morbidity and mortality;

mortality may exceed 10 to 15% in untreated deep vein thrombosis from pulmonary embolus. Proper treatment reduces it to 1%.

Pregnancy is a hypercoagulable state; most pro-coagulant factors, RBC and platelets increase during pregnancy. The following additional physiological changes impose increased risk for TED:

1. Low grade chronic disseminated intravascular co-agulation within the placental bed with deposition of fibrin in the spiral arteries.
2. Venous stasis secondary to uterine enlargement.
3. Placental inhibition of fibrinolysis.
4. Placental separation with subsequent tissue thromboplastin release.
5. Endothelial damage to vessels during operative or vaginal delivery increases maternal thrombotic risk.

Additional risk factors include the following:

1. Previous TED, recent or remote to pregnancy.
2. Preeclampsia or eclampsia.
3. Oral contraceptive drugs.
4. Advanced age, multiparity, obesity, blood group other than O, sickle cell disease.

The problem of pulmonary embolism is two fold:

1. It may present as a complication in patients who are already ill; the manifestations are subtle and diagnosis may be difficult to make. The importance of being certain of diagnosis before starting poten-tially hazardous therapy is evident.

2. Patients may present with acute cardiopulmonary failure. When it appears in the postoperative period the diagnosis is obvious and management is well defined. But the diagnosis is missed, when TED occurs unrelated to surgery, with disastrous consequences.

Sources of Pulmonary Embolism

1. Venous thrombosis in lower limbs
2. Thrombii in right atrium in patients with atrial fibrillation.

The clinical features of pulmonary embolism are due to:

1. Acute circulatory compromise due to obstructed pulmonary circulation resulting in right sided heart failure, pulmonary hypertension and low cardiac output leading to a shock like state.
2. Gas exchange abnormalities characterised by a low PaO_2 with a lowered $PaCO_2$. Arterial hypoxaemia is not very marked (PaO_2 is rarely < 55 mm Hg).
3. Pulmonary infarction may occur, more commonly seen in patients with CHF.

Clinical manifestations are due to poor pre-existing cardiopulmonary reserve, release of vasoactive and bronchoconstrictive substances from platelets; this potentiates pulmonary hypertension, accentuates ventilation-perfusion disturbances and produces tachypnoea.

Clinical Presentation

1. Sudden death.
2. Shock with low output hypotensive state; may or may not be associated with chest pain.
3. Acute right heart failure with increased CVP and neck veins.
4. Acute respiratory failure with dyspnoea, tachypnoea, cyanosis.
5. Acute pulmonary oedema or severe bronchoconstriction.
6. Tachycardia with unstable circulatory state, tachypnoea, fainting or syncope, fall in PaO_2.
7. Pulmonary infarction: Haemoptysis, pleural pain, unexplained pleural effusion in an ill patient suggests embolism.

   Clinical evidence of accompanying venous thrombosis in the lower limbs (tenderness and swelling in calf muscles, tenderness over saphenous vein, rise in skin temperature of one limb) is the strongest indicator of pulmonary embolism.

Diagnosis

Laboratory investigations yield poor and non-specific information. In the high risk settings of thromboembolic disease the following indicate embolic phenomenon:

- Unexplained sudden breathlessness
- Hypoxaemia
- Hypotension.

Investigations

- EKG
- ABG
- X-ray chest (foetus exposed to radiation; should be restricted to select cases)
- Coagulation profile
- Plasma D-dimer
- Impedance plethysmography and Doppler venography.
- Perfusion, scan and pulmonary angiography
- Echocardiography (Transthoracic or Transoesophageal) and pulmonary artery catheterization are more helpful and reliable in excluding other possibilities.

Management

1. Primary therapy with thrombolysis (Streptokinase, Urokinase) and pulmonary embolectomy in massive PTE offers the greatest chance of survival. In acute cases, unfractionated heparin should be started IV and may be replaced by LMWH after several days of effective anticoagulation; treatment is continued during the entire pregnancy and for 4 to 6 weeks, postpartum.

   Heparin 5000-7500 units IV bolus, followed by infusion @ 1000 units/hour. The dose is adjusted to keep the activated partial thromboplastin time (APTT) to about twice the normal value.

2. Temporary inferior vena cava filter can be placed in high risk patients.

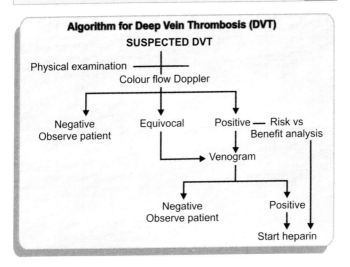

Algorithm for Deep Vein Thrombosis (DVT)

SUSPECTED DVT

Physical examination

Colour flow Doppler

Negative
Observe patient

Equivocal

Positive — Risk vs Benefit analysis

Venogram

Negative
Observe patient

Positive

Start heparin

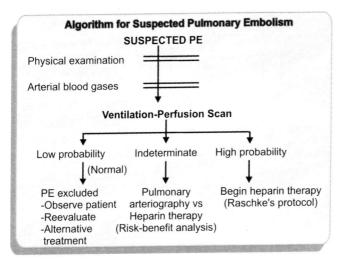

Algorithm for Suspected Pulmonary Embolism

SUSPECTED PE

Physical examination

Arterial blood gases

Ventilation-Perfusion Scan

Low probability
(Normal)

PE excluded
-Observe patient
-Reevaluate
-Alternative
 treatment

Indeterminate

Pulmonary
arteriography vs
Heparin therapy
(Risk-benefit analysis)

High probability

Begin heparin therapy
(Raschke's protocol)

Amniotic Fluid Embolism

Amniotic fluid embolism (AFE) is a rare complication and most cases are fatal despite modern facilities. 10% of maternal deaths from all causes are due to AFE. The pathogenesis of this disorder involves a tear through the amnion or chorion and pressure enough to force the fluid into the venous system; meconium stained amniotic fluid is strongly implicated.

DIAGNOSTIC CRITERIA FOR AMNIOTIC FLUID EMBOLISM

1. Acute hypotension or cardiac arrest.
2. Acute hypoxia (dyspnoea, cyanosis or respiratory arrest).
3. Coagulopathy (laboratory evidence of DIC, severe haemorrhage in absence of other explanation).
4. Acute signs and symptoms occur during onset of labour, Caesarean section, D and C, or within 30 minutes post-partum.
5. Absence of any other significant confounding or potential explanation for signs and symptoms observed.

Management of Amniotic Fluid Embolism

Dopamine, norepinephrine and ephedrine may be useful to maintain blood pressure, but no specific agent is known to be superior to the others in this clinical situation.

Because of the common occurrence of left ventricular failure, inotropic support with digoxin should be considered in nonhypoxic patients.

Pulmonary artery catheterization may provide important information for the clinical management of patients who are hemodynamically unstable.

Pulmonary oedema is very common and must be treated with careful attention to intake and output of fluids.

Corticosteroids may be helpful in the setting of AFE, as the syndrome may be immune mediated; however, the clinical efficacy of corticosteroids is unproven at this time. Hydrocortisone may be administered (500 mg intravenously every 6 hours) until the patient responds or expires.

AMNIOTIC FLUID EMBOLISM

Shock Hypotension	Hypoxaemia	DIC
Monitor CO and BP	Adequate oxygenation	Treat coagulopathy

CPR if indicated	Monitor foetus	Laboratory evaluation
Volume expansion; crystalloid, colloid, blood component Pressor agents: dopamine norepinephrine ephedrine Inotropic agents: digitalis	Increase FIO_2(keep) maternal $PO_2 \geq 60$ mm Hg) face mask; CPAP intubation & mechanical ventilation Pulmonary oedema: furosemide, morphine	Blood component therapy: PRBCs Platelets FFP Cryoprecipitate

Pulmonary artery catheter (if indicated)	Corticosteroids (suggested)	Heparin (controversial)

CO = cardiac output; BP = blood pressure; CPR = cardio-pulmonary resuscitation; FIO_2 = inspired oxygen concentration; ET = endotracheal; DIC = disseminated intravascular coagulation; PRBCs = packed red blood cells; FFP = fresh-frozen plasma; CPAP = continuous positive airway pressure.

Things to be Remembered

- 25% of deaths occur within the first hour of onset of clinical features.
- Abruptio placenta has been the cause in half of the cases of AFE.
- Other predisposing factors are multiparity, older maternal age, overactivity of uterus and overuse of oxytocic drugs, caesarean delivery, IUD, intrauterine foetal or pressure monitoring have been considered potential causative factors.
- Signs and symptoms of AFE are:
    - Sudden desaturation, cyanosis
    - Hypotension, tachycardia
    - Dyspnoea, wheezing, cough, bronchospasm, respiratory distress
    - Chest pain, dysrhythmias, cardiac arrest
    - Headache, unconsciousness, convulsions
    - Coagulopathy (DIC).
- Definitive diagnosis needs demonstration of foetal squamous cells, lanugo hair or vernix in maternal circulation.
- *Management of AFE* requires CPR and immediate delivery of foetus.
    1. Aggressive haemodynamic monitoring (pulmonary artery catheter).
    2. Inotropic support (early).
    3. Oxygenation.
    4. Mechanical ventilation to maintain ventilation and perfusion balance.
    5. Correct the coagulopathy.

VENOUS AIR EMBOLISM (VAE)

Venous air embolism has been seen in normal and caesarean deliveries, removal of retained placenta, in cases of placenta praevia or accreta, in placental abruption, in forceps and vacum delivery; criminal abortions using air, laparoscopy.

Things to Remember

- Sudden and profound hypotension is the most common presenting feature.
- The volume of air that is likely to be lethal varies with rate of infusion of air and patient's position. Any amount greater than 100 ml may be lethal.
- Increased pulmonary resistance and capillary permeability resulting in pulmonary oedema due to infiltrates, lead to acute right-sided failure and hypoxia.

Diagnosis by TEE, precordial Doppler over right atrium, decrease in $EtCO_2$ and increased end-tidal nitrogen. Later on there is increased CVP, hypoxia, hypotension, "mill-wheel" murmur.

Management

1. Stop the procedure, place patient in left lateral decubitus position to trap the embolus in right atrium.
2. Stop further entry of air into circulation by flooding the operative field with saline; if possible, place operative site below the level of the right atrium.

3. If CVP catheter is in place, try to aspirate air from it. Discontinue nitrous oxide.
4. Oxygenation with 100% oxygen helps to remove nitrogen from pulmonary vasculature.
5. Inotropic support with fluids and vasopressors to raise CVP.
6. Mechanical ventilation.
7. Hyperbaric oxygen therapy if available should be used.

Aspiration Pneumonitis

Aspiration is a dangerous and potential lethal problem. During pregnancy, oesophageal sphincter tone is reduced, gastric emptying is slowed and gastric angle is altered leading to increased chances of aspiration; the risk is increased in operative deliveries under anaesthesia, eclampsia, excessive use of narcotics for pain relief and difficult intubation.

Patient may develop symptoms ranging from mild acute lung injury to full fledged acute respiratory distress syndrome. Hypoxia occurs immediately in case of large volumes with solid particles; in cases of small volumes, it may be seen after a delay of 24 hours. Clinical findings are hypoxia, tachypnoea, bronchospasm and diffuse crepts in lungs; presence of shock and severe hypoxia indicate a fatal outcome.

PREVENTION OF PULMONARY ASPIRATION

1. **Reduction of gastric volume**
   Fasting during labour: only small sips of water allowed
   Emptying of stomach by nasogastric tube
   H_2 receptor blockers: Ranitidine
   Metoclopramide
   Omeprazole
2. **Increasing gastric pH**
   Non-particulate antacids: sodium citrate
   H_2 receptor blockers
   Omeprazole
3. **Prevent reflux/regurgitation**
   Metoclopramide (increases lower esophageal sphincter tone)
   Cricoid pressure
4. **Airway protection**
   Regional anaesthesia
   Rapid sequence induction with cricoid pressure
   Rational approach to difficult/failed intubation
   Awake intubation with fiberoptic bronchoscopy.

MANAGEMENT OF ASPIRATION

Trendelenburg position with head turned to side.
Suction upper airways
Place cuffed endotracheal tube
Suction lower airways via endotracheal tube
Administer 100% oxygen, use mechanical ventilation
with PEEP
ABG and continuous pulse oximetry
Chest X-ray
Nasogastric tube to empty stomach contents
Non-particulate antacids
H_2 blocker-Metoclopramide
Beta 2 antagonists to treat bronchospasm
Bronchoscopy to remove particulate matter
Intermittent pulmonary toilet, as needed
Supportive measures as needed (Vasopressors)
Continuous foetal monitoring.

Immediate chest X-ray may not show any abnormality but pulmonary infilterations, mainly radial or prehilar distribution, are seen within 24 to 36 hours.

Majority of the patients show improvement and recovery but 10 to 15% deteriorate and die of respiratory failure within 24 hours; the rest develop various complications such as nosocomial infections, acute respiratory distress and multiple organ failure.

Treatment

1. Oxygenation and antibiotics.
2. Steroids may not be of much help; they suppress neutrophil and macrophage activation and promote secondary infection; currently not recommended.
3. Judicious restriction of fluids helps to improve oxygenation.

Depending upon the severity and extent of acute lung injury, patients may require ventilator support to manage the ventilation and perfusion mismatch.

Cardiogenic Pulmonary Oedema

Valvular cardiac lesions, peripartum cardiomyopathy and myocardial infarctions are important cardiac diseases, which need special consideration during obstetrical anaesthesia practice. Pulmonary oedema, arrhythmias and cardiac failure are serious complications of these cardiac ailments, which get precipitated during pregnancy in third trimester, labour, stress, fluid overload and perioperatively.

Acute pulmonary oedema occurs when fluid transudates from alveolar capillaries into alveolar spaces resulting in foamy transudate in the alveoli, which creates a barrier to oxygenation.

Management includes aggressive monitoring and general principles of pulmonary oedema management:

1. Clearing the alveoli by unloading the pulmonary vasculature.
2. Increasing inspired oxygen concentration.
3. Endotracheal intubation, mechanical ventilation, PEEP.
4. Treatment of the underlying disease process.

TREATMENT OF ACUTE PULMONARY OEDEMA

1. Elevate the head to improve ventilation.
2. Oxygen: Administer via face mask at 10 lit/min or CPAP or endotracheal tube.
3. Furosemide 10 mg/IV, repeat as necessary; maximum of 120 mg in 1 hour.
4. Nitroglycerine, depending on clinical circumstances.
5. Morphine 5 mg IV; avoid in altered consciousness, COPD, increased ICT.
6. Digoxin .5-1 mg IV initially; .2 mg increments 4-6 hours as needed.
7. Continuous foetal monitoring.
8. Mechanical ventilation.

Beta-adrenergic Tocolytic Therapy

Beta-adrenergic drugs (Ritodrine; Terbutaline) are used for treating pre-term labour. β-2 receptor stimulation is needed for tocolysis while β1 activity is associated with unwanted cardiac effects. All beta adrenergic drugs possess some degree of β1 activity.

Tachycardia results from direct stimulation of myocardium (β1effect); there is diminished vascular resistance due to peripheral vasodilatation (β2 effect) resulting in fall in BP with increased cardiac output. Serious complications occur only during prolonged, continuous intravenous use.

Pulmonary oedema is the most serious complication of beta adrenergic therapy, seen after 24 hours of beta agonist infusion, in patients with anaemia, multiple gestation, hypertension, fluid overload and corticosteroid therapy. It is of non-cardiogenic variety, occurring due to capillary permeability defects (seen in maternal bacterial infections). Symptoms are dyspnoea, tachypnoea, haemoptysis and rales; X-ray chest shows alveolar infiltrates. ABG shows increased alveolar-arterial oxygen gradient.

Improvement occurs rapidly after discontinuation of beta-adrenergic therapy.

Treatment of Beta Agonist Complications

Immediate

- Discontinue drug infusion
- Blood pressure support
- Continuous electrography
- Beta blockers
- Treat pulmonary oedema.

Subsequent Care

- Pulse oximetry
- Potassium supplementation
- Calcium supplementation
- Supplemental oxygenation
- Substitute with other tocolytic drug.

Ovarian Hyperstimulation Syndrome (OHSS)

Ovarian Hyperstimulation Syndrome (OHSS) is a serious disorder of unknown pathogenesis due to the use of ovary-stimulating drugs in assisted reproduction programs. Its potentially life-threatening sequelae (due to haemoconcentration) are circulatory shock, ARDS, hepatorenal failure, thromboembolic phenomena, and multiorgan dysfunction syndrome.

Treatment

1. Aggressive resuscitation with low molecular weight dextran and albumin.
2. Close monitoring of central venous pressure, haematocrit, total leucocyte count, electrolytes and blood urea.
3. Clinical classification into mild, moderate, severe, and critical forms of OHSS can help the physician plan appropriate investigations, admission requirements, and acute management.

RESPIRATORY FAILURE IN PREGNANCY

Respiratory failure in pregnancy is a major cause for admission to ICU. It is often a part of complications such as eclampsia, haemorrhagic shock, pulmonary oedema or sepsis. Approximately 0.1% of obstetric patients require controlled ventilation. Maternal mortality is high in these cases.

Causes of Respiratory Failure

1. Pulmonary thromboembolism
2. Amniotic fluid embolism
3. Venous air embolism
4. Aspiration pneumonitis
5. Chest infection
6. Status asthmaticus
7. Pulmonary oedema due to:
    - Cardiac failure
    - Beta-adrenergic tocolytic therapy
8. Pneumomediastinum and pneumothorax following strain
9. Eclampsia
10. Acute respiratory distress syndrome
11. Skeletal abnormalities such as Kyphoscoliosis
12. Morbid obesity.

Multiple factors increase the likelihood of thromboembolic disease during pregnancy such as caesarean section, elderly patient, multiparity, suppression of lactation with oestrogens, obesity and surgery.

Mechanical Ventilation

Acute lung injury results in reduced lung compliance and a marked decrease in the volume of functional lung. Ventilation strategies are designed:

1. To recruit as much lung tissue as possible.
2. Minimising the injurious effects of mechanical ventilation simultaneously.
   - Volotrauma (Alveolar over distension)
   - Barotrauma (High pressure strain to alveolar membrane)
   - Ateletactotrauma (shearing strain because of collapse).

Important Principles

1. Current opinion regarding the optimal technique to ensure adequate gas exchange is to use a low tidal volume with adequate PEEP.
2. The general principles for initiation and weaning of mechanical ventilation in pregnant patients are essentially the same as practiced for non-pregnant patients.

Important Considerations while Dealing Critically Ill Parturient

1. Pregnant females have generalised fluid retention, which shows in tracheal mucosa also. Thus smaller sized endotracheal tube (7.0 mm internal diameter) should be used for tracheal intubation to avoid trauma to mucosa.

2. The goal of ventilation should be to achieve $PaCO_2$ of 30-32 mm Hg (normal values during pregnancy) and PaO_2 of more than 90 mm Hg to ensure oxygenation of foetus. Hyperventilation should be avoided as alkalosis can compromise the oxygen delivery to foetus.

3. Conventional modes of ventilation are used; superiority of any specific mode over others is not yet established. Spontaneous breathing improves patient comfort and recruitment of alveoli, thus should be encouraged. Pressure support ventilation (PSV) and biphasic positive airway pressure (BiPAP) ventilator modes are often preferred in spontaneously breathing patients. Morphine and pancuronium bromide may be used to facilitate tube tolerance and mechanical ventilation.

4. Prop up posture is often used for weaning non-pregnant patients but patients near term may benefit from left lateral position.

5. Automatic tube compensation (ATC) is a new addition to modes of ventilation. This helps to compensate for the non-linearly flow-dependent pressure drop across an endotracheal or tracheostomy tube (ETT) during inspiration and expiration. ATC has been associated with reduced work of breathing, preservation of the natural "noisy" breathing pattern, enhanced synchronisation between the patient and the ventilator, and improvement of respiratory comfort seem to be most important.

6. Nutrition during pregnancy is important for well being of mother and foetus.

- Entral feeding should be preferred over the parenteral feeding. As the pregnant females are at risk of pulmonary aspiration, nasoduodenal tubes are preferred.

- There is a little data available on the use of TPN and proportion of its different components. Fatty infiltration of placenta has been found with use of more than 50% calories as fat. It may be also associated with premature labour.

- Daily allowances of vitamins and minerals should be replenished.

- Glucose monitoring should be done more closely as hyperglycaemia affects the foetus adversely.

SEVERE SEPSIS AND SEPTIC SHOCK

Severe sepsis is an uncontrolled host inflammatory response to infection or tissue injury. Peripartum sepsis is often associated with preterm pregnancies or caesarean sections. Treatment of this syndrome needs:

1. Early and aggressive removal of source of infection
2. Management of physiological derangements associated with this syndrome.

The most common causative organisms are beta haemolytic streptococci, *Escherichia coli* and *Staphylococcus aureus*. Most microbes were found to be susceptible to first- or second-generation cephalosporins in one of study. Treatment of peripartum sepsis with second-generation cephalosporin is usually effective and the outcome is good.

Management

Diagnosis

In postpartum period fever along with the following signs and symptoms, indicate severe sepsis and septic shock.

- Unexplained tachycardia, tachypnoea, hypotension
- Decreased urine output
- Elevated leucocyte count and serum lactate levels

Prior to starting antibiotics obtain 2 or more blood cultures. At least one blood sample should be withdrawn from a fresh site and one may be from a venous site placed more than 48 hours earlier. Other samples include urine, tracheal and surgical wound swabs.

Initial Resuscitation

Begin resuscitation immediately in patients suspected to have sepsis.

Resuscitation goals are:

- Central venous pressure: 8-12 mm Hg
- Mean arterial pressure > 65 mm Hg
- Urine output > 0.5 ml/kg/hr
- Mixed venous oxygen tension > 70% if monitored.

If there is failure to achieve central venous or mixed venous oxygen tension more than 70% with CVP of more than 12 cm H_2O, then transfuse RBCs to achieve a haematocrit of > 30%, or administer a dobutamine infusion (Maximum dose 20 microgram/kg/min).

Antibiotic Therapy

Begin antibiotic therapy as soon as sepsis is recognised. Administer one or more drugs that are active against the likely bacterial or fungal pathogens. Consider microorganism's susceptibility pattern. Reassess antimicrobial therapy for neutropenic patients and those with pseudomonas infections. Stop antimicrobial therapy immediately if the condition is found to be non-infectious.

Source Control

Evaluate patient for a focus of infection and need for dilatation curettage of uterus or exploratory open drainage. Choose source control that will result in minimal physiological derangement and will be sufficient to accomplish the goal. Remove intravascular access devices or central venous catheters that are a potential source promptly after establishing fresh vascular access at other sites.

Fluid Therapy

Resuscitate with crystalloids or colloids. Achieve central venous pressure of 10 cm of H_2O or give a fluid challenge of 500-1000 ml of normal saline or 300-500 ml of colloids, if there is no central venous pressure monitoring. In case of positive response, fluid therapy is instituted at slower rate till adequate perfusion and urine output is achieved.

Vasopressors and Inotropic Therapy

- Start vasopressors to achieve adequate arterial blood pressure (Systolic pressure > 90 mm Hg) till tissue perfusion is restored by fluid resuscitation.
- Although dobutamine infusion is better for septic shock, low blood pressure may preclude its use in initial resuscitation.
- Either norepinephrine or dopamine administered through a central venous line is the initial vaso-pressor of choice.
- Consider dobutamine infusion once adequate blood pressure is achieved. Do not increase cardiac index to achieve an arbitrarily predefined level of oxygen delivery.
- Role of low dose dopamine for renal perfusion and as diuretic is no more recommended.
- Consider vasopressin in patients refractory to fluid and conventional inotropes and vasopressors.

Vasopressors, Inotropes and Inodilators

Drug	Dose range	Remarks
Dopamine	< 2 μ/kg/min (diuretic dose) 2-10 μ/kg/min (predominantly β) 11-20 μ/kg/min (predominantly α)	Effect is dose-dependent
Dobutamine	2-20 μ/kg/min	
Dopexamine	0.5-6 μ/kg/min	Has predominant beta 2 effects
Noradrena-line	0.02-2 μ/kg/min	Vasoconstrictor
Phenyle-phrine	0.2-1 μ/kg/min	Vasoconstrictor
Vasopressin	0.01-0.04 units/min	Vasoconstrictor
Milrionone	Loading 50 μ/kg Infusion 0.3-0.75 μ/kg/min	Inodilator
Enoxamine	Loading 0.5-1 μ/kg Infusion 5-20 μ/kg/min	Inodilator

Steroids

- Treat patients who fail to respond to fluid, vaso-pressors and inotropic therapy, with steroids.
- Hydrocortisone 200-300 mg/day, in divided doses or by infusion is given for 7 days. Decrease steroid

dose if septic shock resolves and taper off at the end of therapy.

- Do not use steroids to treat sepsis in the absence of shock unless the patient's endocrine history or steroid therapy history warrants it.

Recombinant Human Activated Protein C

- RhAPC is recommended in patients at high risk of death.
- Main indications are multiorgan dysfunction syndrome with two or more organ involvement.
- Dose schedule 100 units /kg over 72 hours in central venous line preferably.
- Bleeding tendencies contraindicate its use. It is contraindicated for 3-4 days in the postoperative period.

Other Supportive Therapies

Blood and Blood Products

- In the absence of significant cardiac disease or acute haemorrhage, transfuse packed cells or whole blood to raise haemoglobin to a target value of 7gm/dL.
- If there is evidence of clinical bleeding or patient has to undergo invasive intervention, transfuse FFP (10-15 ml/kg) or 5-7 units.
- Transfuse platelets if count is less than 5000/mm^3, or counts are between 5000-30,000/mm^3 but there is significant risk of bleeding, when patient has to

undergo surgery (Target value is $>50,000/mm^3$, $>100,000/mm^3$ preferred).

- Do not use erythropoietin to treat sepsis related anaemia.
- Do not transfuse FFP to normalise measured values of PTI or APTT.

Mechanical Ventilation

- Mechanical ventilation may be required in patients developing sepsis related Acute Lung Injury (ALI) or ARDS.
- Prefer spontaneous modes of ventilation over the modes having minimum mean airway pressure to prevent haemodynamic instability.
- Use larozepam or narcotic sedation, depending upon whether patient needs additional analgesia or not.
- Avoid neuromuscular blocking drugs.

Glucose and Parenteral Therapy

- Enteral therapy is always better than parenteral therapy.
- Prefer low energy and low protein TPN protocol to prevent catabolic process but provide sufficient calories for sepsis.
- Maintain glucose levels < 150 mg/dL (8.3 mmol/L) using glucose and insulin infusions.
- Bicarbonate therapy is not recommended unless pH is less than 7.10.

302 STEP BY STEP ANAESTHESIA IN OBST AND GYN

Renal Replacement

Continuous venovenous haemofiltration or intermittent haemodialysis depending upon haemodynamics of patient and dialysis indications.

DVT Prophylaxis

- Low molecular weight heparin or unfractionated heparin can be used if there is high risk of DVT
- Use mechanical compression devices in cases where heparin or LMWH is contraindicated.

Stress Prophylaxis

H_2 receptor antagonists or Sucralphate 1 gm 6 hourly.

SUGGESTED READING

1. Dellinger RP, Carlet JM, Masur H, et al. Surviving Sepsis Campaign guidelines for management of severe sepsis and septic shock. Crit Care Med 2004;32(3):858-73.

Chapter 24

Cardiopulmonary Resuscitation of the Pregnant Patient

Cardiopulmonary arrest is uncommon (occurring once in every 30,000) during pregnancies. Resuscitation-guidelines have been developed principally for sudden death from ischaemic heart disease, which is rare during pregnancy. The unpredictability and rarity of cardiac arrest during pregnancy make any preparation difficult. The single most important factor in improving the survival chances of mother and baby is an organised time-conscious team approach.

The Reasons for Cardiorespiratory Collapse in Pregnancy

Accidents, pre-eclampsia, eclampsia, hypertensive heart diseases, sickle cell disease, complication of tocolytic therapy, complicated epidural analgesia, drug toxicity or hypersensitivity, pulmonary embolism, amniotic fluid embolism, peri-partum haemorrhage with hypovolaemia, water intoxication, prostaglandin administration, ischaemic heart diseases, pre-existing cardiac diseases, e.g. cardiomyopathies and special situations such as drug abuse, septic shock and HELLP syndrome.

Effect of Pregnancy on Cardiopulmonary Resuscitation

Pregnancy produces physiological changes, which during maternal cardiac arrest make it more difficult to resuscitate the mother.

1. It is a high cardiac output state (increase by 150%) with increased blood volume with low systemic vascular resistance and low colloidal oncotic pressure. Uterus receives 30% of cardiac output.

2. Enlarging uterus imposes changes on the respiratory system:
   - Upward displacement of diaphragm reduces FRC (functional residual capacity).
   - Reduced FRC with increased oxygen demand in pregnant women leads to reduced arterial and venous oxygen tension.
   - Minute ventilation (MV) increases due to effect of progesterone.
   - Increased MV results in maternal respiratory alkalosis; there is increased renal excretion of CO_2 by the foetus. Hence increase in maternal CO_2 (as seen in cardiac arrest) will lead to foetal acidosis.
   - Mother compensates for hypoxia by reducing uteroplacental blood flow, which may cause foetal distress.

In later half of pregnancy, aortocaval compression by gravid uterus renders resuscitation more difficult because of:

1. Decreasing venous return (upto 30% of blood volume).
2. Supine hypotension.
3. Decreasing effectiveness of thoracic compressions.
4. Obstruction to forward flow of blood when blood pressure is low (as seen during cardiac arrest).

Other obstacles in effective resuscitation are:

1. Vasopressors used in resuscitation cause utero-placental vasoconstriction leading to reduced foetal oxygenation and CO_2 exchange.
2. Reduced GIT motility and reduced tone of lower oesophageal sphincter result in increased risk of aspiration of gastric contents.

CARDIAC ARREST TEAM

Cardiopulmonary arrest in the labour and delivery area tends to be a chaotic event. It is imperative that there be an organised team approach with tasks performed in a time conscious manner. The team will have, at minimum, these members:

- Team leader
- Airway person
- Chest compression person
- Vascular access person
- Drug preparation person
- Drug administration person
- Event recorder
- Obstetrician to perform caesarean delivery
- Neonatologist/paediatrician.

Each individual on the team should understand his or her particular assignment. The equipment needed is that which is necessary to sustain ACLS, to perform caesarean delivery and to resuscitate the newborn infant. It is the responsibility of the team leader to direct team members according to the situation and to be aware of the duration of cardiac arrest.

Pathophysiology of Cardiopulmonary Arrest in Pregnancy

Maternal cardiopulmonary arrest results in maternal and foetal hypoxia due to the sudden decrease in oxygen supply. The uteroplacental unit is responsible for the exchange of the gas between mother and the foetus. Foetal tissue oxygen supply depends on maintenance of adequate gas delivery from mother. Because of the changes that take place during pregnancy, maternal systemic and uterine oxygen delivery exceeds the minimal level necessary to sustain maternal and foetal life. During cardiopulmonary arrest, oxygen delivery to the maternal tissues and the uterus is markedly reduced or eliminated completely. There are no maternal or foetal adaptations to such severe reductions in oxygen supply that allow maintenance of tissue viability; tissue death begins in minutes.

Goals of Cardiopulmonary Resuscitation (CPR) during Pregnancy

The principal goal of CPR is to restore spontaneous breathing and circulation as quickly as possible. Once a stable rhythm is achieved, emphasis is placed on maintaining adequate oxygen delivery, so that both maternal and foetal oxygen consumption can be maintained The precipitating event leading to cardiopulmonary arrest during pregnancy is difficult to determine at the time of arrest. It is helpful to consider the arrested pregnant patient as having a severe form of shock, often with moderate or severe hypoxaemic lung disease. In non-pregnant patients, chest compression results in cardiac output equal to approximately 30 % of the normal. In late pregnancy, the supine position results in decreased venous return (due to inferior vena cava compression by the gravid uterus) resulting in reduced cardiac output. It follows that,chest compression in a pregnant patient, in supine position will result in even more drastic decrease in cardiac output and oxygen delivery to maternal tissues. Additionally, compression of aorta by gravid uterus results in decreased uterine blood flow and therefore decreased foetal oxygen delivery. It is recommended that during CPR, manual displacement of uterus to the left be attempted or place the patient in 15 to 30 degrees left lateral tilt position; this, however, makes chest compression more difficult to perform and less effective.

Management

CPR may be needed outside or inside the hospital. Logically the chain of survival approach should be followed. This includes early CPR, early defibrillation, early advanced care and early stabilisation.

OUTSIDE THE HOSPITAL

Basic and advanced life support in the form of rescue breathing, chest compressions, and Automated External Defibrillators (AEDs) should be used.

In case of Foreign Body Airway Obstruction (FBAO), chest (sternal) thrust and finger sweep of the mouth should be used instead of abdominal thrust (Heimlich manoeuvre).

For airway protection, use cricoid pressure during ventilation to prevent aspiration.

Chest compressions should be performed displacing the uterus away from the great vessels; this is done by manual lifting of the uterus or wedging the body by pillows under the right side of the abdomen.

INSIDE THE HOSPITAL

- Basic CPR along the lines of ABC is initiated.
- To prevent gastric aspiration, early endotracheal intubation is done.
- Immediate caesarean section is indicated if the mother is not revived within 5 minutes. Delivery of the baby is associated with better prognosis, both for the mother as well as the baby.

TREATMENT OF DYSRHYTHMIAS

- Follow the standard algorithm for the type of arrhythmia recorded. The new American Heart Association algorithm stipulates the use of DC shock and drugs in CPR.
- Both elective cardioversion and emergency defibrillation can be used with success in pregnant women.

- Foetal arrhythmias due to electrical induction by defibrillator can be minimised by proper placement of the paddles. The left breast should be should be pushed out of the way and wide posterior paddle is used, if available.

ANAESTHETIC CONSIDERATIONS

Patients with cardiac problems:

- Patients with valve prosthesis are at increased risk of cardiac trauma when closed chest cardiac compression is used; so open chest cardiac compression be considered. When ever patient with severe cardiac disease is electively taken up for surgery, cardiac surgery team along with the perfusionist is informed, since cardiopulmonary bypass (femoral artery-vein bypass) may be life saving.

Local Anaesthetic Toxicity

Bupivacaine is 10 times more cardiotoxic than lidocaine. It has a strong affinity for myocardial tissue and its action will last for hours. A large IV dose (accidental) will cause asystole due to its effect on conducting system and contractile myocardial cells. If CPR fails in this situation, immediate caesarean section is warranted, since the foetal heart may also be affected. The use of open chest CPR and then cardiopulmonary bypass to treat local anaesthetic toxicity has been successfully carried out.

MODIFICATIONS IN CARDIAC CARE OF PREGNANT PATIENTS

1. Left uterine displacement: Manual, use of Wedge, tilt of table.
2. Aggressive airway management—intubate early.
3. Delivery within 5 minutes if foetus is viable.
4. Aggressive restoration of circulating volume, if needed.
5. If standard doses of drugs are ineffective, consider using higher doses because of expanded plasma volume due to pregnancy.

KEY INTERVENTIONS TO PREVENT ARREST

1. Place pregnant patient in left lateral position (or manually displace the uterus).
2. Give 100 % oxygen.
3. Give a fluid bolus.
4. Immediate re-valuation of the drugs being administered.

Basic Life Support (BLS) Modifications during Arrest

Relieve aorto-caval compression by manually displacing the uterus, or placing a wedge (pillow) or placing the back of the patient on the rescuer's thigh, or tilting the operating table.

Flow chart 24.1

Cardiopulmonary arrest

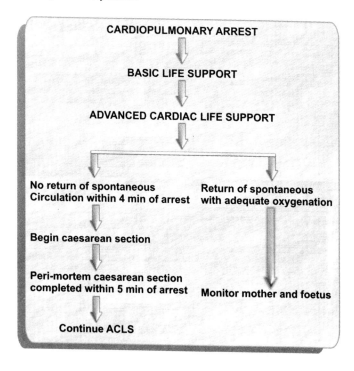

Advanced Cardiac Life Support (ACLS) Modifications during Arrest

Consider possible aetiologies, e.g. magnesium sulfate toxicity.

If the above procedures fail to revive the patient consider immediate peri-mortem caesarean section.

Involve the obstetrician and the neonatologist when possible.

Peri-mortem Caesarean Section

It is performed to save the life of the foetus and the mother. The baby has the greatest chance of being healthy, if delivered within 5 minutes after the mother's cardiac arrest. Also that the mother's cardiovascular function improves dramatically after the delivery of the foetus, probably due to relief of aorto-caval compression. The recommendation is to complete the delivery of the baby by emergency caesarean section no more than 5 minutes after spontaneous maternal circulation ceases. Memory Aid: "The Four-Five Rule" Begin the perimortem caesarean section 4 minutes after the mother's cardiac arrest to have the baby delivered no later than 5 minutes after cessation of spontaneous circulation.

SUMMARY

Goals of CPR-ACLS
1. Establish stable rhythm
   Drugs
   Cardioversion
   Electrical pacing
2. Maintain oxygen delivery
   (cardiac output × oxygen content)

Cause	Treatment
Cardiogenic	Drugs
Hypovolaemic	Fluids

Obstructive   Airway/oxygen
Distributive   Chest compression

PREGNANCY CPR (IDEAL)

1. ACLS should benefit both mother and baby.
2. Foetal monitoring should be available.
3. Continue ACLS and deliver baby to improve maternal and foetal survival.

PREGNANCY CPR (REALITY)

1. Cardiac arrest is a rare event during pregnancy.
2. Precipitating event is often difficult to identify.
3. Difficult to predict mother's response to ACLS.
4. Foetal monitoring is difficult.
5. Need to make time dependant decisions for foetal-maternal viability.
6. Not much data available on CPR on pregnant patients.

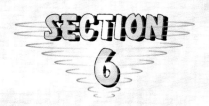

SECTION
6

MISCELLANEOUS

Chapter 25

OT Errors and Accidents

"Too err is human"
"There is always scope to improve."

The theory of planned behaviour is applicable to every skilled individual and specialty; the anaesthetists are no exceptions. Common violations of safety guidelines by the anaesthetists include failing to visit patients preoperatively, failure to perform pre-anaesthetic equipment checks and silencing of alarms during anaesthesia.

Facts

1. Anaesthesia related death rate is 1/500 developing countries as compared to 1/70000 in developed countries.
2. Avoidable mortality rate is 3 to100 times higher in developing countries.
3. Equipment misuse is three times more frequent than equipment failure.
4. Multiple sequential errors result in a mishap.
5. Human factor contributes to 80% of cases, directly or indirectly.
6. System to be emphasised rather than individual to prevent errors and mishaps.
7. Main factors:
   - Poorly trained personnel.
   - Absence of, or poorly maintained equipment.

Common Problems

1. Airway or ventilation related problems resulting in hypoxic brain injury or death.
2. Erroneous drug administrations.

Common Components of Problems

(In decreasing order of frequency)
1. Breathing circuit
2. Vapourisers
3. Ventilators
4. Medical gas lines
5. Anaesthetic machine
6. Monitors.

Common Pitfalls

- Fresh gas flow hypoxic mixture.
- Gas leaks.
- Excessive anaesthetic agent.
- High airway pressures.
- High inspiratory carbon dioxide.
- Ventilator malfunction and mis- or disconnection of patient circuit.
- Failure of intubation equipment.

Common Hazards/Mishaps

1. Hypoxia
2. Pollution of OT
3. Arrhythmia

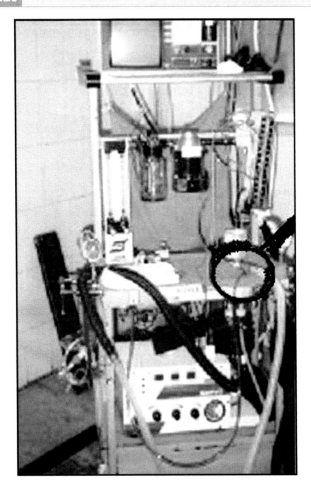

Figure 25.1

Showing misconnection of Bain circuit tubing with ventilator tubing resulting in increase in dead space ventilation and hypercarbia in a patient

4. Barotrauma
5. Awareness
6. Infection
7. Explosion/fire.

HOW TO PREVENT EQUIPMENT ERROR

- 'Push and twist' to check male-female connections.
- Always, if you turn the ventilator off, keep your finger on the switch.
- Use monitors and alarms, but eternal vigilance is the key.
- Use apnoea alarms and don't silence them.
- If the ventilator fails:
  1. Manually ventilate with the circle system.
  2. If 1 is not possible, then bag with oxygen (if a portable cylinder is available) or room air.
  3. If 2 is not possible, then try to pass suction catheter through the tracheal tube.
  4. If 3 is not possible, then visualise the hypo-pharynx and cords, or reintubate.
- Get proper and quality anaesthesia and monitoring equipment.

HOW TO PREVENT DRUG RELATED ERROR

1. Avoid long working hours as fatigue and stress lead to error in judgment.
2. Conscious checking of drug label.
3. Labelling of filled syringes.

The protocol with mnemonic "*COVER ABCD*" by Runciman's et al. (*Runciman, et al. Errors, incidents and accidents in anaesthetic practice. Anaesth Intens Care 1993;21:506-09*) is helpful to remind the steps for prevention of error.

C Circulation, Color

O Oxygen, Rota meter

V Vapourizer, ventilation

E Endotracheal tube, examination anaesthesia machine

R Re-evaluate; Review other equipment

A Airway—for laryngospasm, obstruction

B Breathing—for bronchospasm, pulmonary oedema, collapse, pneumothorax

C Circulation

D Drugs—For wrong dose, wrong drug.

No error–No accident–No death–No loss

Chapter 26

Legal Issues

With implementation of consumer protection act to medical services, the medicolegal suits have increased over last the decade in India. Services provided by anaesthesiologists have been the subject matter of judicial review time and again. The Consumer Disputes Redressal Commissions/Forums have defined services of an anaesthesiologist and also what is and what not 'deficiency' in the services is:

Service

Section 2(1) (0) of the Consumer Protection Act 1986 defines the word service. 'Service' means service of any description which is made available to potential users and includes the provision of facilities in connection I with banking, financing, insurance, transport, processing, supply' of electrical or other energy, board or lodging or both, housing construction, entertainment, amusement or purveying of news or other information but does not include the rendering of any service free of charge or under a contract of personal service. The Supreme Court has held that the services provided by the medical fraternity falls within the ambit of the word 'service' as defined by Section 2(1) (o) of the Consumer Protection Act 1986.

Deficiency

The word' deficiency' has been defined by Section 2(1) (g) of the Consumer Protection Act 1986. "Deficiency"

means any fault, imperfection, short coming or inade-
quacy in the quality, nature and manner of performance
which is required to be maintained by or under any
law for the time being in force or has been undertaken
to be performed by a person in pursuance of a contract.
Thus failure to provide standard desired service by an
anaesthesiologist is deficiency. This deficiency includes:

1. Negligence and rashness—Lack of caution and
   requisite care, absence of anaesthesiologist during
   transfer.
2. Contributory negligence—Patient not telling the pre-
   existing medical disease to anaesthesiologist,
   otherwise which would have avoided the problem,
   per se diabetes mellitus.

   Negligence can amount from civil to criminal
depending upon the act.

Civil negligence (malpractice): When plaintiff accuses the
doctor in civil court for carelessness or poor care or
wrong diagnosis or poor standard of care.

Criminal negligence: It is grave situation. It means doctor
has shown gross mistake and has been rash in executing
the duty amounting to near death or resulting in death
of patient. This is non-bail able offence and negligent
act amounting to homicide under section of 304-A of
IPC.

Standard of Care

An anaesthesiologist must possess and exercise
reasonable degree of skill and knowledge, but not

highest expert skill at the risk of being found negligent. It is a well established law that it is sufficient if he exercises ordinary skill of an ordinary anaesthesiologist exercising that particular art. The court will accept the expected errors and mistakes on the part of anaesthesiologist even when working against time or dire stressful situations taking in "Risk benefit ratio".

Accepted Practices

Is level of skill and care practiced by peer anaesthesiologists.

Informed Consent

Informed consent means as a consent of patient or his attendant when he is incompetent to give consent, to his medical practioner prior to rendering service by him, provided that medical practitioner has explained about the procedure and it's Sequa in his vernacular language. Absence of consent is liability, but its presence is not a license to be negligent.

Blanket consent given at the time of admission does not suffice for the operative procedures.

There are ever changing answers for a lot of questions about informed consent such as:

- Who should take consent, doctor or his assistant?
- Where and when to take consent?
- What should be told or not?
- How much should be revealed about the procedure and complications?

- What to do in emergency?

The justified answer to all these queries is to tell the patient that enough what should make him to understand the situation to make wise decision and should not get scared of. In emergency situations life saving procedure may be performed and patient/ attendant may be told later after completion of procedure with details of grave situation you faced to take such an urgent decision.

Deviation from Accepted Practice

Deviation from accepted practice is negligence if anaesthesiologist fails to justify the deviation; otherwise error of commission is not negligence.

Accidents

Accidents or mishaps are not punishable. Doctor is not liable if, a treatment which in ordinary circumstances would be safe, but has resulted in unforeseen adverse effects, per se an anaesthetic drug has resulted an anaphylaxis and death, which is normally not expected and doctor has taken due precautions also.

Error of Judgment

An error of judgment in itself is not negligent act.

Inherent Risks

Every procedure has its own inherent risk for which an anaesthesiologist cannot be liable.

Discretion of Anaesthesiologist

Anaesthesiologist has the choice to use discretion when there are more than one ways of treating a particular problem. Anaesthesiologist is supposed to tell the patient of various options available prior to start anaesthesia such as regional/general anaesthesia.

Vicarious Liability

Hospital is liable for the act or services of anaesthesiologist or employees. Consultant is responsible for the work done by his subordinate or resident doctor who is under trainee.

Deficiencies in Statutory Requirements

Required qualification and registration with State Medical Council or MCI is essential.

Generally speaking it is for the plaintiff to prove negligence of defendant (doctor) who is otherwise presumed innocence except in a condition called 'Resipsa loquitar'—it speaks for itself, e.g. hypoxic brain damage after disconnection of breathing circuit or ventilator.

Chapter 27

Obstetric Anaesthesia Practice Guidelines

(Adapted from a report by the American Society of
Anaesthesiologists Task Force on Obstetric Anaesthesia)

In era of evidence based practice, guidelines and recommendations are necessary clinical tools to make decision in various clinical situations. These practice guidelines also help in risk-management protocols in routine, complex and critical situations. In addition these guidelines provide directions for medical research and educational tools. Practice guidelines are not standard or absolute requirements.

PREANAESTHETIC EVALUATION

- Focus on history and examination related to maternal health and anaesthesia related obstetric history, an airway examination and baseline blood pressure record.
- Examine back for feasibility of regional block.
- In case of significant risk factor, the problem should be discussed with concerned obstetrician.
- Intrapartum platelet count: A specific platelet count for regional block has not been determined. Platelet count may be ordered in individual cases on the basis of clinical relevant history and examination or signs of coagulopathy.
- Blood type and screen: Although blood typing is done in all obstetrical patients for obstetrical reasons, but may be ordered by anaesthesiologist also, e.g. if there is anticipation of bleeding.
- Foetal heart rate (FHR): FHR should be monitored by a qualified personnel prior to and after administration of regional block for painless labour.

FASTING STATUS

Clear Liquids and Solids

- Modest amount of clear fluids may be taken by un-complicated labouring patients (fruit juices without pulp, carbonated drinks, clear and black coffee).
- Type of fluid is more important than the volume of fluid.
- Patients at higher risk of aspiration and surgical delivery should be restricted to oral intake on individual case-to-case basis.
- Solids should be avoided in labouring patients. A specific fasting time for solids that is predictive of anaesthetic complications has not been determined.

ANAESTHESIA CARE FOR LABOUR AND VAGINAL DELIVERY

- Anaesthesia care is not essential for all parturient during labour.
- Maternal request for painless delivery is sufficient justification to provide pain relief during labour, but the selected analgesic technique depend on the medical status of the patient, progress of labour and the facilities.

Epidural Analgesia

- The literature supports the use of epidural analgesia compared to parentral opioids.

- The literature indicates that low concentrations of epidural local anaesthetic combined with opioids are associated with lesser incidence of motor blockade as compared to higher concentrations of local anaesthetics alone.
- Appropriate resources and back up should be available to treat complications (respiratory arrest, hypotension, nausea vomiting, and pruritus).
- Epidural infusions should be preferred over single bolus injection for painless delivery.

Spinal Opioids with or without Local Anaesthetics

- The literature is equivocal regarding analgesic efficacy of spinal opioids and epidural local anaesthetics.
- Rapid onset of spinal analgesia has advantageous over epidural local anaesthetics and may be used in advanced labour in selected patients.

Combined Spinal and Epidural Analgesia

Task force recommends that CSE may be used to provide rapid and effective labour analgesia.

Regional Analgesia and Progress of Labour

- Task force recommends not to use cervical dilatation as a means of determining timing of regional analgesia, rather recommends deciding timing on individual basis.

- Epidural analgesia may be used for previous caesarean section without adversely affecting the incidence of vaginal delivery.

Monitored Anaesthesia Care

Monitored or stand by Anaesthesia care should be made available whenever requested by the obstetrician.

REMOVAL OF RETAINED PLACENTA

- Regional/general anaesthesia may be used depending upon the haemodynamic status of the patient
- Nitroglycerine is an alternative to terbutaline or general anaesthesia with halogenated agents for tocolysis during removal of retained placental tissue.

ANAESTHESIA FOR CAESAREAN DELIVERY

- The literature suggests that a greater number of maternal deaths occur when general anaesthesia is administered.
- The consultants agree that regional anaesthesia can be administered with fewer maternal and neonatal complications and improved maternal satisfaction when compared to general anaesthesia.
- The decision to use a particular technique should be individualised case to case based on several factors (elective vs. emergency, patient preferences, anaesthesiologist's choice, haemodynamic status).

- Resources for management of complications (airway, hypotension, nausea, vomiting, inadequate anaesthesia, pruritus) and resuscitation should be available.

POSTPARTUM TUBAL LIGATION

- Both consultants and task force agree that spinal, epidural and general anaesthesia can be used safely for postpartum tubal ligation, preferably after eight hours of delivery.
- Task force recommends assessing the patient's haemodynamic and fasting status for anaesthesia risk and feasibility of a particular technique.

MANAGEMENT OF COMPLICATIONS

Resources for Management of Bleeding Emergencies

1. Large IV bore catheters
2. Fluid warmer
3. Forced air body warmer
4. Blood bank services
5. Rapid infusion devices.

Suggested Equipment for Airway Emergencies

1. Rigid laryngoscope blades and handles of alternative design and sizes. The task force believes fibreoptic intubation equipment should be available.
2. Endotracheal tubes of assorted size.

3. At least one device suitable for emergency non-surgical airway ventilation (retrograde intubation, a hollow jet ventilation stylet, cricothyroidotomy kit and combitube/laryngeal mask airway).
4. Endotracheal tube guides.
5. Equipment suitable for emergency surgical airway access.
6. Topical anaesthetics and vasoconstrictors.

Central Invasive Haemodynamic Monitoring

The data is insufficient to indicate whether advanced haemodynamic monitoring is associated with reduced incidence of complications. The decision to have or have not should be individualised on case to case basis.

Cardiopulmonary Resuscitation

Basic and advanced life support facility should be available in labour and delivery units.

Appendices

Appendix 1: MAC of Inhalation Agents

Anaesthetic agent	MAC
Nitrous Oxide	104
Halothane	0.75
Enflurane	1.66
Isoflurane	1.15
Sevoflurane	2.0

Appendix 2: Local Anaesthetic Agents

Drug	Minimum effective concentration	Max. dose (Plain)	Max dose (with 1 in 200,000 adrenaline)
Lignocaine	0.25%	200 mg	500 mg
Bupivacaine	0.175%	150 mg	150 mg
Ropivacaine	0.25%	250 mg	Not yet defined
Prilocaine	0.5%	400 mg	600 mg

Appendix 3: Intravenous Agents used in Anaesthesia

Drug	Dose	Repeat dose/Infusion rate
Thiopentone	5-6 mg/Kg	2 mg/Kg
Propofol	1-3 mg/Kg	0.5 mg/Kg
Methohexitone	1.5 mg/Kg	0.5 mg/Kg
Etomidate	0.2 mg/Kg	0.1 mg/Kg
Ketamine	1.5-2 mg/Kg	0.5 mg/Kg Infusion: 40 µg/Kg/min
Diazepam	0.1-0.3 mg/Kg	
Midazolam	0.05-0.1 mg/Kg	
Flumazenil	0.1-0.5 mg	
Fentanyl	0.025-0.1 mg	Infusion 4-10 µg/Kg/h
Alfentanil	5-10 µg/kg	Infusion 05.-10 µ/Kg/min
Sufentanil	0.1 µg/kg	Infusion 0.01 µ/Kg/min
Succinyl choline	1-1.5 mg/kg	Infusion 4-10 mg/min
Pancuronium	50-100 µg/kg	
Atracurium	50 µg/kg	Infusion 0.5 mg/Kg/h
Vecuronium	100 µg/kg	Infusion 0.2 mg/Kg/h
Mivacurium	150-250 µg/kg	
Pipecuronium	50 µg/Kg	
Neostigmine	30-80 µg/Kg	
Edrophonium	0.2-1 mg/Kg	
Pyridostigmine	50 µg/Kg	

Appendix 4: Vasoactive Drugs

Drug	IV bolus	IV infusion	Duration
Adrenaline	20-100 mcg (hypotension) .5-1 mg (cardiac arrest)	.5-4 mcg/min	1-2 min
Noradrenaline	xxxxx	1-30 mcg/min	1-2 min
Dopamine	xxxxx	2-10 mcg/kg/min	5-10 min
Dobutamine	xxxx	2-30 mcg/kg/min	5-10 min
Esmolol	.25-.5 mg/kg	50–200 mcg/kg/min	10 min
Nitroglycerine	50-100 mcg	.1 mcg/kg/min	4 min
Nitroprusside	xxxxx	.2 mcg/kg/min and titrate	4 min

Appendix 5: Agents Producing Neuromuscular Blockade

Agent	Initial dose (mg/kg)	Duration (min)	Elimination	Associated effects
Depolarising				
Succinylcho-line	1.0-1.5	3-5	Plasma cho-linesterase	Fasciculations, increase or decrease in heart rate, hyperkalaemia, known malignant hyperthermia
Nondepolarising				
Mivacurium	0.15	8-10	Plasma cholin-esterase	Flushing, decrease in BP
Atracurium	0.2-0.4	20-35	Ester hydrolysis	Histamine release
Cisatracurium	0.1-0.2	20-35	Ester hydrolysis	
Vecuronium	0.1-0.2	25-40	Primarily hepatic	
D-Tubocurare	0.5-0.6	75-100	Primarily renal	Histamine release, decrease in BP
Pancuronium	0.04-0.1	45-90	Primarily renal	Increase in heart rate, mean arterial BP, and cardiac output
Doxacurium	0.05-0.08	90-180	Primarily renal	Decrease in BP

BP = Blood pressure

Appendix 6: Monitoring Standards During Surgery

Essential

1. Continuous presence of appropriately qualified anaesthetist
2. Oxygen supply failure alarm
3. Continuous monitoring of cardiac output
4. Observation of reservoir bag and chest excursion
5. Ventilator disconnect alarm
6. Oxygen analyzer of inspired gases
7. Electrocardiogram
8. Non-invasive arterial blood pressure.

Strongly Recommended

9. Spirometry
10. Pulse oximetry
11. Temperature
12. End-tidal carbon dioxide
13. Monitoring of neuromuscular blockade.

Appendix 7: Preanaesthetic Machine Check

At the beginning of the session

1. Check the controls 'off'.
2. Check gas supplies, both cylinder and pipeline.
3. Inspect and check function of:
   a. Oxygen supply failure alarm
   b. Oxygen/Nitrous oxide ratio protection
   c. Oxygen flush
   d. Mechanical ventilator and disconnect alarm
   e. Waste gas scavenging system.

Before each case

1. Check reserve Oxygen supply.
2. Check function of breathing system.
3. Check vapouriser.
4. Check absorber, if in use.
5. Inspect equipment for:
   • Endotracheal intubation
   • Intravenous infusion
   • Resuscitation.
6. Check function of high vacuum suction apparatus
7. Apply and check monitoring systems
8. Set appropriate alarm levels.

Appendix 8: Estimation of Intraoperative Fluid Loss and Guide for Replacement

Preoperative deficit	Maintenance IVF × hr npo, plus preexisting deficit related to the diseased state
Maintenance fluids	Maintenance IVF × duration of case
Third space and insensible losses	1-3 ml/Kg per hr for minor procedure 3-7 ml/Kg per hr for moderate procedure 9-11 ml/Kg per hr for extensive procedure
Blood loss	1 ml blood or colloid per 1 ml blood loss **or** 3 ml crystalloid per 1 ml blood loss

Appendix 9: Calculation of Maximum Allowable Blood Loss

$$\text{MABL} = \frac{\text{EBV} \times (\text{Starting haematocrit - Target haematocrit})}{\text{Starting haematocrit}}$$

MABL = Maximum allowable blood loss
EBV = Estimated blood volume

Appendix 10: Routine Preoperative Testing

Test	Comment
Complete blood cell count	Possibility of substantial blood loss, patients with chronic illnesses
Urinalysis	Urologic symptoms, instrumentation of the urinary tract, possibility of surgical placement of prosthetic materials
Serum electrolytes, creatinine, and blood urea nitrogen	Patients > 60 yr, diuretic use, chronic diarrhoea, renal disease, liver disease, diabetes
Coagulation studies	Family history of bleeding disorder, patient history of abnormal bleeding, anticoagulant usage, liver disease
Biochemical profiles (including enzymes)	History of liver or biliary disease liver
Pregnancy testing	Any woman of childbearing age (except posthysterectomy patients)
Chest X-ray	Risk for pulmonary complications, thoracic or cardiac procedures
Electrocardiogram	Women > 50, history of cardiovascular disease or arrhythmia, diabetes
Blood type and cross/type and screen	Type and screen if risk of substantial blood loss is low; type and cross if moderate risk of substantial blood loss

Appendix 11: Potential Indications for Preoperative Pulmonary Function Tests

- Heavy smoking history
- Chronic cough or severe exertional dyspnoea
- Morbid obesity
- Neuromuscular or chest wall disease

Appendix 12: Risk Prediction in Abdominal Surgery

Parameter	Normal	Mild risk	Moderate risk	High risk
FVC	> 80% of predicted	50-80%	30-50%	< 1 L (25-30%)
FEV_1	> 80% of predicted	1-2 L	0.5-1.0 L	0.5-0.6 L (25i-30%)
FEV_1/FVC	70-78%	40-65%	30-45%	< 30%
MVV	> 80% of predicted	50-80%	35-50%	< 35%
$PaCO_2$	35-40 mm Hg	40-45 mm Hg	40-45 mm Hg	> 45 mm Hg

FEV_1 = Forced expiratory volume in 1 second;
FVC = Forced vital capacity;
MVV = Maximum voluntary ventilation

Appendix 13: Delivery System

Type	FIO₂ capability	Comments
Nasal cannula	24-48%	At flow rates of 1-8 L/min. true FIO₂ uncertain; dependent on minute ventilation; simple, comfortable.
Simple face mask	35-55%	At flow rates of 6-10 L/min
High humidity mask	28-100%	Flow rates should be 2-3 times minute ventilation; excellent humidification
Reservoir mask (non breathing)	90-95%	At flow rates of 12-15 L/min;
Partial rebreathing	50-80%	At flow rates of 8-10 L/min;
Ventimask	available at 24%, 28%, 31%, 35%, 40%, 50%	Provide controlled FIO₂; useful in COPD poorly humidified gas at maximum FIO₂

FIO_2 = Fraction of inspired oxygen

Appendix 14: Factors affecting Position of Oxyhaemoglobin Dissociation Curve

Left shift (Increased affinity)	Right shift (Decreased affinity)
Alkalosis	Acidosis
Hypocarbia	Hypercarbia
Decreased temperature	Increased temperature
Decreased 2,3 DPG	Increased 2,3 DPG
Hypophosphataemia	
Banked blood	
Sepsis	
Carbon monoxide	

Appendix 15: Physiologic Definition of the Appropriate Level of PEEP

Best PaO_2
Best A- a O_2 gradient
Intrapulmonary shunt = 15%
Best dynamic compliance (V/P)
Best Oxygen transport ($CaO_2 \times CO$)
Best mixed venous oxygen content

Appendix 16: Arterial Blood Gas

Normal values:
- PaO_2 > 75 mm Hg
- SaO_2 > 95%
- $PaCO_2$ 36–44 mm Hg
- pH 7.36–7.44
- $[H^+]$ 40 ± 4 mEq/L
- $[CO_2]$ or $[HCO_3]$ 24 ± 2 mEq/L

Appendix 17: Nutritional Requirements

	Requirement
Water	25-35 ml/Kg/day
Proteins	1 g/Kg/day
Carbohydrate	2 g/Kg/day
Fat	1-2 gm/Kg/day
Calories	30 Kcal/Kg/day

Appendix 18: Strength of Solutions

- 0.1% solution contains 1 mg/ml
- 0.5% solution contains 5 mg/ml
- 1% solution contains 10 mg/ml

A drug concentration expressed as ratio is converted as follows:

- 1:1000 = 1 gm/1000 ml = 1 mg/ml
- 1:10,000 = 1 gm/10,000 ml = .1 mg/ml
- 1:1,000,000 = 1 gm/ 1,000,000 ml = 1 mcg/ml
- 1 mg = 1000 micrograms (mcg)
- 1 ml = 16 to 18 drops of regular drip set
- 1 ml = 60 drops of micro drip set

Appendix 19: Conversion Factors

Millimoles/litre = mg/litre divided by molecular weight
1 mm Hg = 1.36 cm H_2O = 0.133 kPa
1 cm H_2O = 0.098 kPa
1 kPa = 7.5 mm Hg = 10 cm H_2O

Appendix 20: Modified Ramsay Sedation Scale

Score	Characteristics
1	Anxious and agitated or restless, or both
2	Cooperative, oriented, and tranquil
3	Responding to commands only
4	Asleep, but responds to physical or auditory stimuli
5	Asleep, but responds sluggishly to physical or auditory stimuli
6	No response

Appendix 21: Normal Values

Haematology	Reference range
Haemoglobin	13-18 gm/dl
Total leucocyte count	3,900-11,000/cu mm
Differential leucocyte count	
Neutrophils	40-75%
Lymphocytes	20-45%
Monocytes	0-10%
Eosinophils	0-6%
Basophils	0-1%
Absolute eosinophil count	
Platelet count	40-400/cu mm
Reticulocyte count	1.5- 4.5 lakhs/cu mm
ESR (Westergren)	.2-2%
Bleeding time	0-20 mm in first hour
Clotting time	2-5 minutes
Prothrombin time	4-10 minutes

Biochemistry

Blood sugar	
Random	60-180 mg/dl
Fasting	60-110 mg/dl
Postprandial	90-140 mg/dl

Liver Function Tests

Serum bilirubin	upto 1 mg/dl
Direct	0-.3 mg/dl
Indirect	0-1 mg/dl
SGOT	8-33 IU/L
SGPT	4-36 IU/L
Alkaline phosphatase	20-130 IU/L
Total proteins	6-7.8 mg/dl
Albumin	3.2- 4.5 mg/dl
Globulin	2.3-3.5 mg/dl

Contd...

Contd...

Haematology	Reference range
A:G ratio	1.2-2.2
Serum amylase	< 120 IU
Serum lipase	< 190 IU

Renal Function Tests

Blood urea	15-40 mg/dl
Serum creatinine	0.5-1.1 mg/dl
Serum uric acid	2.7-7.3 mg/dl

Electrolytes

Serum sodium	135-150 mEq/L
Serum chloride	95-195 mEq/L
Serum potassium	3.5-5.3 mEq/L
Serum calcium	8.5-11 mEq/L
Serum magnesium	1.2-2.2 mg/dl

Lipid Profile

Total cholesterol	< 200 mg/dl
Triglycerides	< 190 mg/dl
VLDL	< 40 mg/dl
LDL	< 130 mg/dl
HDL	> 35 mg/dl

Index